A Way Back To
Health

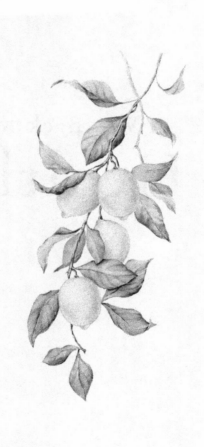

A Way Back To
Health

12
Lessons
from a
Cancer Survivor

Kelley Murray Skoloda

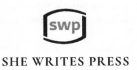

SHE WRITES PRESS

Published 2021
Printed in the United States of America
Print ISBN: 978-1-64742-217-2
E-ISBN: 978-1-64742-218-9
Library of Congress Control Number: 2021912126

For information, address:
She Writes Press
1569 Solano Ave #546
Berkeley, CA 94707

Interior design by Tabitha Lahr

She Writes Press is a division of SparkPoint Studio, LLC.

To David, the wind beneath my wings.
To Jake, Ellie, Mom, Colby, and the other
angels who helped me through many unexpected
lessons on my journey with cancer.

Contents

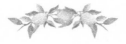

Foreword

Acancer diagnosis doesn't come with a how-to manual or a blue-print on how to cope with this instantly life-changing ill-ness. What it does offer is the opportunity to learn and benefit from people who have tread a similar path before you.

As I read the manuscript of this book, I often found myself saying out loud, "That's right," or, "I wish I had thought of that!" I could easily relate to Kelley's experiences and appreciate her lessons learned even though my surgery and treatment were for breast cancer.

At the heart of this book is a truth that sounds simple. It is "Be your own advocate. Do what feels right for you." Caught up in the fear of the unknown and the often-rapid march from diagnosis into surgery or treatment, it is easy to lose sight of your own inner strength and voice. This was true for me.

Like Kelley, I rediscovered my power when I started to take better control of the things that I could. I became active in managing my care, I took advantage of the days that I felt better after chemotherapy to reconnect with family and friends, and I learned how to listen to my body and focus on what was important to help me heal.

When I finished treatment, I became determined to empower other women to have a better-prepared, well-informed, "take-charge" recovery. Women coping with all forms of cancer. I cofounded my company Cancer Be Glammed to educate and enable them to reclaim their lifestyles and to recover with dignity, positive self-esteem, and personal style.

For the past ten years I have been immersed in the cancer world—a world that is ever-changing. The one constant throughout has been the amazing resilience, heart, and generosity of the doctors, nurses, caregivers, survivors, and their families that share their hard-won wisdom to support other people traveling this difficult road.

I have never felt like "cancer is a gift," but I have come to believe that the people it brings into your life are.

Lisa Lurie
survivor, author, and cofounder
Cancer Be Glammed
www.CancerBeGlammed.com

Introduction

I was the healthiest person I knew until I became a cancer patient. As a child, my grandmother and mother prepared meals at home. We rarely ate out, in part because of expense, but mostly because my family liked to cook in the Italian tradition of food equating to love. The food was delicious and nutritious—handmade pastas and soups—made from fresh ingredients from my Pap's garden. I have continued many of these traditions throughout my adult life: buying fresh, local produce for my family, cooking most meals at home, avoiding fast food, taking nutritional supplements, and eating as healthy as possible.

My dad was an athlete in his younger years—fast enough to go to state competitions in track. I followed in his athletic footsteps, starting my athletic career as an eight-year-old gymnast. Gymnastics and then track filled my elementary and high school years, and I earned eight letters for sports. By the time I went to college, running, lifting weights, and coaching gymnastics were routine parts of my life. As an adult, aerobics, weightlifting, skiing, golfing, yoga, meditation, and a generally active life were my norms. Even while working in an office setting for several decades, I always belonged to a gym and attended classes regularly. For God's sake, my triceps weren't even super jiggly!

Doctor's visits were rare occurrences, except for an occasional flu, yearly checkups, and pregnancy-related checkups. Even when I was pregnant, my health remained fully intact. While three months pregnant with my son, our first child, I climbed the Great Wall of China. The day before my son was born, I worked out on our at-home stair climber hours before going into the hospital to give birth. I gained twenty-five pounds with my first pregnancy and thirty with my second and lost all the baby weight within six months of delivery.

That's why when I went in for my first routine colonoscopy, I was anxious (who isn't when someone is about to stick a camera up your butt?) but not expecting anything out of the ordinary. No symptoms, no sickness, a lifelong healthy lifestyle. What could possibly go wrong?

I was the healthiest person I knew until the day of my colonoscopy.

I had no idea colorectal cancer was incredibly common. When I asked my doctor how, given my lifestyle, eating, and exercise routines, I could have colon cancer, he said that my only risk factor was how common colon cancer now is.

According to the American Institute for Cancer Research, colorectal cancer is the third most common cancer worldwide, the third most common among men, and the second most common among women. Who knew? There were over 1.8 million new cases in 2018. And the problem is getting worse. The global burden of colorectal cancer is expected to increase by 60 percent to more than 2.2 million new cases and 1.1 million deaths by 2030.[1] Unfortunately, chances are pretty good that you or someone you love will encounter colorectal cancer.

For many years, fifty was the recommended age for a first colonoscopy screening. However, in 2018, the year I was diagnosed, the American Cancer Society released updated guidelines for colorectal cancer screening. Among the major guideline changes, the new recommendations say screening should begin at age forty-five, for people at average risk. The ACS lowered the age to start screening after analyzing data from a major study. The numbers showed that new cases of colorectal cancer are occurring at an increasing rate among *younger* adults. After reviewing this data, experts on the ACS Guideline Development Committee concluded that a beginning screening age of forty-five will result in more lives saved.[3] In October 2020, the United States Preventive Services Task Force (USPSTF) announced plans to lower the recommended colorectal cancer screening age to forty-five for individuals of average risk, which will certainly save lives.

Being familiar with the statistics and the updated guidelines provides strong rationale to encourage screenings. In my experience, however, there is nothing like a personal story to provide real motivation, which I learned in a powerful way when I first shared my story.

On June 5, 2018, a week after my colectomy surgery, I was recovering at home. The diagnosis had been life changing, and I felt the need to let my friends and business network know what had happened. Through an article on *Medium* (which can be found in its entirety in the Appendix of this book) and a Facebook post, I shared the story of my situation, diagnosis, and surgery. At that point I did not yet know that chemotherapy treatment would soon be in my future.

As a result of sharing my story, I was soon inundated with not only well wishes but also reactions like "I've been meaning to schedule my colonoscopy screening and now I'm doing it," and "Your story has incentivized me to get my [husband/mother/father] scheduled for their next screening." Dozens and dozens of people responded and were taking action, not because of the new guidelines (which had just been released and in the news that week), but because of a personal story.

Despite how much the story seemed to help others, I went into stealth mode during the next treatment phase of chemotherapy. While I felt the need to publicly share the first part of my story, I felt an even stronger need to keep the rest of the story secret, until now.

Cancer is ugly. It sounds cliché until you go through it, but it is really ugly. Physically, every system in my body was affected. The treatments are toxic. The side effects are sickening and relentless. I couldn't eat, sleep, digest, poop, or live normally. The doctors' appointments are time-consuming, and the healthcare system is maddening to navigate. The anxiety and mental anguish infiltrate daily life and impact everyone in the family. While I was a regular at the chemo infusion center, losing weight rapidly and suffering toxic side effects, I didn't want "cancer" to take over my life. So only my family and very closest friends knew what I was enduring.

I still wrestle with sharing my story because I don't want the pain of reliving even a second of the ugliness. But what I have found is that there is pain in *not* sharing a part of my life that has forever changed who I am. A relentless researcher and avid reader, I've also learned so many lessons that could be helpful to others that I feel compelled to share.

After undergoing the full process, from diagnosis to surgery to chemo and back to health, I learned a great deal along the way. I witnessed other patients and their families struggling with challenges like I had experienced. They are lessons I never wanted or expected to learn, but they helped me and, based on the power of personal stories, could help others who are coping with a similar situation.

Being a professional marketer and storyteller by trade and having previously published a business marketing book, the idea of writing a book about my cancer experience was almost second nature, though the idea of reliving the stories was scary. Sometimes writing the story was too painful and I had to walk away. Other times, the feeling of survival and a drive to share what could be helpful to others would win. In the end, what I learned was too compelling for me to keep to myself because I didn't know then what I do now and too many people are in the same situation.

This book contains "lessons" in key areas that capture and detail the learning. Each lesson represents an area of unexpected learning for me and contains background, statistics, and my personal perspectives, as well as those of other cancer survivors. Through the power of personal stories, the lessons are meant to help people advocate for themselves or a family member as they wrestle with cancer and its treatment.

You'll see that I tell my personal story in chapter one so that as we move through the lessons you'll have a frame of reference. Parts of my personal story are also embedded in each chapter. The stories share my feelings and emotions about what I was experiencing at the time. These experiences led to the discovery of my unexpected lessons.

In talking with other survivors, I found that many share similar sentiments. To explore an even wider range of experiences, my editor suggested that I incorporate lessons from other cancer survivors. My "call for survivor stories" on Facebook and LinkedIn received an amazing response. Fellow "warriors" shared moving and powerful stories with me and granted me permission to share them in this book.

While reading the stories shared with me, I felt like my immense pain and suffering paled in comparison to what so many others and their families, especially children, have endured.

There is such a quiet strength among these survivors. Like me, many people choose to not share their journey publicly and suffer privately. Given the ubiquity of cancer in general, someone you know is likely suffering right now, and there is always someone who is having a worse day than you.

I approached the lesson chapters mostly from a chronological-progression perspective. However, after reading the first foundational chapter, the lesson chapters can be read in any order that is most meaningful or useful to the reader. You'll find my personal experiences and advice coupled with the stories of others, as well as some facts and data embedded into each lesson chapter.

I am still not sure why God chose this path for me. While I figure that out, perhaps my journey can serve as a guide to ease the suffering for others through self-advocacy and, perhaps, as a catalyst for much-needed changes in our healthcare system.

I remain positive that everything will be OK, and I still believe that I am the healthiest person I know. With so many blessings and so many lessons learned, some of which I'll share with you in the next chapters of this book, my hope is that someone can take away some learning that can help them or a loved one should cancer strike. I also hope that medical professionals—especially oncology doctors and nurses—can see from this first-person account how they impact patients' lives.

Please let me know your thoughts and experiences as we work together to share personal stories that will help others to combat cancer and survive cancer treatment.

Contact me at www.awaybacktohealth.com.

CHAPTER 1:

My Story

*There is no greater agony than bearing
an untold story inside you.*
—Maya Angelou

When I awoke in the dark at 5:30 a.m. that Friday in late April, it was predicted to be a beautiful spring morning. *Just another day.* My stomach was growling a bit from the colonoscopy prep— no food and almost twelve hours of "cleansing"—and no food or drink allowed that morning. "The prep is the worst part," they all say. Despite the prep, I was determined that I could make it a few more hours when I'd come home after a clean bill of health, eat a hearty breakfast, and enjoy an early start to a nice weekend.

My husband drove me the short ten minutes to the outpatient surgical center where the colonoscopy procedure would be done. My mom, a retired nurse, would meet us there. Never a fan of medical procedures, I was quiet and a bit tense on the ride, but my husband's chatter and pleasant demeanor kept things light.

Going into the procedure I had done my homework, wanting to know what my body would go through. I talked in advance to the anesthesiologist to ensure that I would not be given any opioids, not wanting to have any addictive drugs in my system. Not one to take medication, I didn't like the idea of anesthesia. But clearly, this is a necessary evil when a scope is to be inserted in your ass-end and up into your colon.

Pulling into the parking lot at the surgical center, I was happy to see only a few cars. I had purposely scheduled the first appointment so I could be in and out quickly. Check-in was routine with a short wait in the reception area and then back to the changing/pre-procedure holding area. The nurses who greeted me were pleasant and made me feel comfortable.

After answering the long series of questions about my health—do I smoke, no; drink, no; take any medications, no; have any symptoms of any kind, no; and on and on and on, always no—the nurse commented that my remarkably healthy lifestyle was rare and my procedure would be over before I knew it. Soon after changing into the procedure gown and lying down on the hospital bed, the IV line was inserted into the top of my hand for the anesthesia. As soon as the anesthesia started, I dozed off within seconds.

It felt like only a few minutes had passed when I heard my name being called. Still in a fog, I felt a twinge of pain, like a slight menstrual cramp. Always sensitive to the tones of people's voices, my intuition signaled that something wasn't right. Slowly, my mind responded to the call and I began to come to my senses. Still under the influence of the anesthesia, I could hear the doctor saying things like "large polyp," "need to send for testing," and "I can recommend a surgeon and oncologist."

What the hell is she talking about?

What does that mean? An appointment with an oncologist, a full-on cancer doctor?

As we prepared to leave, the doctor indicated that the polyp was unusually large and could be cancerous. It was likely to be colon cancer.

What?

How could this be? It was impossible. I did nothing that would cause this. I did everything to prevent such a thing. I had no symptoms. Yet here I was. The polyp was to be biopsied, and the results of the biopsy would be available "early next week."

Do I really have to wait that long to know if something bad is happening?

Waiting was cruel and unusual punishment. I had family, work, and more business travel to tend to. I didn't have time for such a bump in the road.

Still dazed, I said goodbye to my mom, and my husband and I left the surgical center and got into our car. We were both completely shocked. In the past hour, without any notice, our world was basically turned upside down and inside out. My husband, always positive, assured me that everything would be OK while I cried and stared at the car floor, my head in my hands in disbelief. Despite how often we hear or read the word "cancer," hearing the word associated with yourself is devastating and inconceivable. And fear. I had so much fear. The fear was so real and scary that it took my breath away and made me sick to my stomach. The fear took me to a place I'd never known before.

Over the course of the day, reality sank in. I sat on the couch in my family room in a state of both extreme sadness and disbelief. The kids were at school, so I openly cried to try and get all my emotion out before they came home. I would try to be as normal as possible for the kids until we knew for sure. My son was getting ready to graduate from high school, and we had so many happy events to celebrate in the next few weeks, including my daughter's dance recital.

The weekend seemed to never end, and I was incredibly sad for most of it. I waited. I cried. I tried to think positively. And then I cried and waited some more.

The results were in on Monday, and the news was not good. The polyp was cancerous. While it was removed, there was no way to tell if the cancerous cells had penetrated the cell walls of my colon. To make this determination I needed a CT scan and to consult with a surgeon for a procedure called a colectomy.

What the hell is a colectomy?

A colectomy is an operation where a part of your colon is removed. How much needs to be removed is determined by your diagnosis. That diagnosis is aided by first having a CT scan.

While the CT scan was an easy procedure physically, I was a nervous wreck going into the scan the following Friday. I was told the CT results would be processed quickly. And they were. I called the GI doctor's office at three o'clock that Friday, as instructed, and the results were in. The doctor, however, was not. They said the results couldn't be shared. I asked for the doctor to call me anytime, and as soon as possible.

Saturday came, no call back.

Sunday came. Same.

When Monday came I called the office again, first thing in the morning. I was anxious and crying and about out of my mind. I was crazy.

"The doctor is off on Mondays," the receptionist said.

Are you freaking kidding me?

I asked for the doctor's mobile number. I explained the circumstances, again, and asked for a call back. No call back.

Tuesday morning came, and I finally got the call from the GI doctor who did my colonoscopy and ordered the further tests.

"Your colon appears clear."

Relief.

"However, there is no way to know definitively, and surgery is still the recommended course of treatment. Also, the CT scan showed multiple nodules in your lungs and a nodule in your left breast."

I couldn't breathe.

In addition to going to see a surgeon for a colectomy, I would now need to quickly get a diagnostic mammogram for potential breast cancer and get a second CT scan with a focus on my lungs.

All of this may sound confusing, and, in fact, it was so incredibly confusing that it made my head spin. One doctor's appointment, opinion, and test led to another, and another; I felt like a used car that went in for a regular oil change and came out needing a new exhaust system, new tires, and another appointment to check the engine.

Before meeting with the surgeon about the colectomy, I went to my ob-gyn to get direction for a follow-up diagnostic mammogram. I was in a state of high anxiety. The ob-gyn's office had artwork on the walls as many do. All the artwork featured Greek architecture. But in the treatment room where I was seen, there was a single butterfly photo taped to the wall. The taped butterfly was so random, but I took it as a positive sign that my breast and lung issues would resolve.

I entered a several-week phase of almost constant doctors' appointments after my colonoscopy. Going to appointments was a full-time job, and I already had a full-time job as well as a family to take care of. Time blurred. Priorities shifted. I was at the mercy of my condition and doctors' schedules. We waited and waited and waited in waiting rooms.

One of the most emotionally trying aspects of this phase was the retelling of my diagnosis and condition, over and over again, to nurses, admins, residents, and doctors. It was almost a disincentive to getting a second opinion, but on the positive side, I was encouraged to become my own advocate and record-keeper.

I had lost some trust in my gastrointestinal doctor because she had delayed so long in communicating to me about my CT scan, but I still met with her recommendation for a colectomy surgeon. Several other reliable sources recommended the same surgeon. He reviewed my results and, indeed, recommended a colectomy. In his office, I was a mess. I was a puddle of tears, nerves, and uncertainty. Even though medical qualifications were a top priority to me, the unsatisfactory answer to a silver-bullet question suggested by a surgeon friend made me decide to seek a second opinion.

"Can I have your cell phone number?"

"I don't give out my number," he said.

I pressed. "If I really feel I need it, would you provide it?"

"If you really need it," he said.

When I got home, I kept thinking about my talk with the doctor and discussed it with my husband. It didn't feel right. But time and "cancer" pressure weighed heavily on me. Finally, I talked with some close family and friends and received a referral from my sister, who is exceptionally well-versed in the healthcare system due to my nephew's health challenges. The doctor she referred me to worked out of a much larger health system, one that had a great reputation for medicine but not so much for personal attention.

Feeling like a second opinion was necessary before deciding, I called the surgeon's office. The efficiency was apparent from the first call. When I explained my circumstances, an appointment was made within a week. The office worked to get all my medical records into their system in advance of me seeing the surgeon. There is a lot to be said for comforting medical care, but when in a serious health situation, efficiency is even more welcome.

The day of the appointment, my husband, mom, and I were at the Starbucks in the hospital, and my mom spotted a nurse in front of us in line with a surgical cap that was covered with butterflies (my sign). She remarked that even as an operating room nurse for forty years, she had never seen a surgical cap with a butterfly motif.

The waiting-room time was brief, and the surgeon was prepared. He had already looked at the colonoscopy results and all my other tests. He was personable, and he performed multiple colectomy surgeries *almost every day*. They could slot me in for surgery the day after Memorial Day, and he and his chief resident would check on me every day while in the hospital. This all felt good to me.

I was a bit more in control of myself this round and asked my same list of questions. The recommended course of treatment was identical. I could have easily stopped there and gone with the first surgeon, who was in a more geographically desirable location. But with my prepared questions as my guide, I pressed on. Finally, I got to my silver-bullet question.

"Can I have your cell phone number?" I asked.

"Of course," he said, and he wrote it down on a piece of paper. He also provided me with a "back office" number so I could immediately reach nurses.

While I labored a bit over the decision, I knew in my heart the decision was made.

Along with spending dozens of hours in hospitals and doctors' offices, I did my own research and homework on my condition. They say you should never search the Internet when you're sick, but doing my own research made me well-informed. In fact, I was even asked if I was a healthcare professional.

The thought of major surgery in a month scared me out of my mind. I tried to stay calm and upbeat. Except for my nearest family and a handful of close friends, no one knew my situation. My daughter's dance recital would be four days after my colectomy surgery, and getting to see her dance became a guiding beacon as I went into surgery. While most people are in the hospital for five days for a colectomy, I talked myself into getting discharged in four to make that recital.

There were many moments in between when I just wanted to crawl into a hole and cry. Much like with my pregnancies, though, I decided that if I went into the surgery in great shape, I'd come out in decent shape. So I spent the month working out like a fiend and eating as nutritionally as I could. I prayed. I meditated. And then Memorial Day came—a holiday most celebrate with food—and I had to bowel prep. I would not be allowed to eat for four days. Hamburgers, hot dogs, and all food was off-limits.

Feeling like I had been gone for days, I heard my voice being called in the distance. I tried to pull myself out of another anesthesia-induced haze. My husband and mom were in the room. It was hard to communicate. As I started to regain my capacities, I realized that my abdomen was hugely swollen and that I was hooked up to an IV infusion as well as a catheter. I felt like a truck had hit me.

Ice chips were the only thing I could eat or drink. After a few hours, water was allowed. I was so thirsty—and hungry. Food was not allowed until my bodily functions started to work again, which means I needed to pee and then poop. Given I could not even get out of bed, it was hard to imagine that such a time would come. A liquid diet was the interim step.

Having anticipated that hospital food would be bad-tasting but not necessarily bad for me, I made my own chicken-broth soup and brought it to the hospital with me. Instead of the sugar- and salt-laden liquid tray they tried to give me, I ate my own soup, which the nurses kindly kept in a nearby refrigerator and heated for me.

Three days after I got home from the hospital, my surgeon's cell number popped up on my phone. Expecting a check-in, I picked up the call and was excited to tell him I was making good progress. He was happy to hear of the progress, and he had the pathology results to share. I honestly assumed everything was fine and that I'd just need to recover and move on.

This was not the case.

My colon was indeed clear. *Amen.* But the complete pathology was not OK. As is standard procedure, he removed nearby lymph nodes as well. Removal of twelve nodes is standard. He removed twenty-six, a substantial sampling. Of the twenty-six, twenty-five were clear, but one had cancerous cells.

Shit.

Walking into a building called a "cancer treatment center" is one of the most humbling and disconcerting experiences I have ever had. I'm sure the nice elderly greeter, who kindly directed us to the elevator, understood this when I started bawling in response to his direction. Arriving in the waiting room was truly shocking. It was packed! Every chair was full and people were standing. The prevalence of cancer and related statistics popped up in my reading often, but seeing the real-life impact hit me like a revelation.

After checking in with the receptionist, the admin for my assigned pod, and the vital-stats nurse, we waited for the doctor. The resident came in first and, once again, I shared my whole long and painful story. Then I shared my story with the physician's assistant, who informed me chemotherapy would be the recommended course of treatment.

Um, what? Chemo?

Maybe I had been overly optimistic or maybe I had ignored the cold hard truth, but when she said the word "chemo," I lost it. How could I possibly be someone who needed chemo?

I was the healthiest person I knew.

The oncologist was a reputable, knowledgeable straight shooter with a quirky sense of humor—a survival skill in the cancer world. He talked about drugs with long, hard-to-pronounce names, names that now role off my tongue effortlessly. Mostly he talked about statistics, which blew me away. Call me a fool, but based on all those hospital and medical ads that talked about personalized medicine, I had thought my treatment would be based on me, not just numbers. But the truth was that cancer is a numbers game. Surgery cures the problem 75 percent of the time. Chemo improves your odds by another 9 to 10 percent.

Given I was young and healthy, the recommendation was to proceed. How I was to proceed was based on statistics—this time, clinical trial statistics. My treatment would be based on what had been tested and proven to work on others, mostly others who did not resemble me at all. A two-part chemo regimen was recommended—infusions of oxaliplatin (a platinum-containing compound) every three weeks, coupled with an oral chemo drug, Xeloda (capecitabine). Fortunately, this regimen had recently been reduced to three months, instead of six months, based on a recent clinical trial.

Still, I had so many questions. What are the side effects? How sick will I get? Can I care for my family? Work? Will I lose weight? Lose my hair? Lose my mind?

Once the regimen was decided, I opted to have the actual treatments at a local extension of the cancer center, which would decrease my travel time significantly. Having had surgery just a few weeks before, it was much more difficult to physically get in shape, as I had done before surgery. Walking, at first just around the house and then more extensively in my neighborhood, was about the only exercise my body could endure.

Before treatment could start, insertion of a port was recommended. A chemo port is a round medical device, about the diameter of a half-dollar coin and about a half inch thick. It's surgically implanted into the chest, most often, and used as a port for IV infusion needles because the chemo can be very hard on your veins in a traditional IV setup. It was described to me as "a quick outpatient procedure."

Bah.

More like another painful, time-consuming, and temporarily life-changing procedure that left me feeling like I had a stack of half dollars embedded in my chest, protruding so significantly that I could not even look at it in the mirror without my stomach turning.

Walking into the chemo center for the first time was difficult. Still in disbelief, I had a hard time keeping it together. I wanted to cry anytime anyone said anything to me. I was struck by how many people were there to be treated. The waiting room was full and, as I came to find out, the treatment area was nearly filled to capacity every single day. I had no idea so many people were suffering from cancer and undergoing chemo right in my area.

The pervasiveness of cancer is crazy.

Some kind nurses prepped me physically and with information before the chemo infusion. Steroids and antibiotics were administered through the port. Then the flow of what I considered to be toxic liquid started. At first, I felt OK. Then a little weird. My heart rate raced a little and my head buzzed. The entire process lasted nearly four hours.

I went home, worked, and had dinner, and though I felt strange, I managed. The oral medication was also started that same day. Two pills in the morning, two at night, for two weeks. I came to think of them as poison pills. The medication made me tired and suppressed my appetite and my energy, but I could still eat a bit, work, and walk daily.

I began to experience unrelenting diarrhea, lack of appetite, food aversions, oral neuropathy, and a lack of physical strength that left me all but unable to walk—all things disturbingly common with chemo and that also contributed to significant weight loss. When I explained my side effects to my nutritionist and told her I was trying to remain on anti-inflammatory foods, she looked at me like I had three heads. She then recommended drinking Ensure and putting butter on everything. *This is the best nutritional advice you can give?* She then proceeded to give that same advice to pretty much every other patient in the infusion center.

As I underwent chemo, I researched the clinical trials and white papers. The patient demographics usually skewed older, which was obvious since about 90 percent of the people in the infusion center were much older than me. I couldn't help but wonder if the chemo regimen I was on was right for me. If I was so sick after three weeks,

I couldn't imagine what patients thirty years older than me were experiencing.

The third week, my week off, was supposed to be better. It wasn't. In fact, it was much worse, and when the big problems with side effects kicked in, the side effects became so intense that I created a "calendar of pain and suffering" to track them: waves of almost unbearable digestive tract pain and diarrhea that made eating almost impossible and dictated that I be close to a bathroom at all times; a reaction to cold that turned simple things like reaching into the refrigerator or going to the grocery store into painful experiences; and huge blisters on my feet that made it impossible to wear shoes. Every smell or scent bothered me. I stopped grocery shopping, cooking, eating, and walking. I took my daughter to school and worked. That was pretty much it.

I also called my local oncologist's office to tell them about the horrible level of multiple side effects. "That's to be expected" was the advice I received. I went through with my second round of IV and oral treatment. The symptoms got even worse. I became plagued with almost constant diarrhea, which ended up lasting nearly three weeks. I called the doctor's office repeatedly asking what I should do. "This is to be expected. Take Imodium as directed." When I asked to have my doctor call me back personally, I was told he does not like to talk to patients on the phone.

I continued to work and go to meetings. In fact, I was running meetings. Several times I thought I'd keel over from the pain while I was speaking. Finally, I simply could not go on in the condition I was in. I knew my body could not take any more, physically or mentally. I called the doctor's office and insisted that he call me back. He finally called at 5:00 p.m. the next day. I described my situation, the side effects, and how long they had lasted. He said he was not previously aware of my condition and that my side effects were on the 99 percent mark of the bell curve for severity.

No shit. That's pretty much what I had been saying for three weeks to his office.

I also called the oncologist who originally prescribed the course of treatment, not the one who wouldn't return my call, and went to meet with him again. His reaction when I told him my story was to say, "We failed you."

A pause in the chemo was recommended for as long as I needed to get my body back in physical condition to receive treatment. Plus I would need a reworked treatment plan. I would immediately start IV fluids, several times a week, to restore what I had lost through weeks of diarrhea. The IV infusion drug would be reduced and given every two weeks, and the oral chemo med was reduced as well.

After a three-week break, I resumed treatment. This time around I was assigned a nurse to monitor my treatment and side effects. She was fantastic—proactive, responsive, and on top of every detail. I was also assigned an IV infusion nurse, who always gave me my fluid and chemo infusions. She was also fantastic—caring, knowledgeable, and gentle.

I did what I could do each day and focused on the time, posttreatment, when I should start to feel better—in my case, Thanksgiving and Christmas. Eating the best turkey dinner became a goal. Buying concert tickets for a show in December—at the height of chemo toxicity—reminded me that I'd get there.

Finally, in early November, after four torturous months, I had my last infusion. When I was done, my fantastic infusion nurse and the other nurses gathered round me. They handed me some bells.

"These are for you to ring. They're the 'end of chemo' bells," she said.

I rang them and cried.

The moment took my breath away.

CHAPTER 2

Learn to Trust Your Instincts

Have your own experience and trust your intuition. A million people will tell you what you should and shouldn't be doing, but you know yourself and your body best—do what you think is right.

—CHRISTINA STEINORTH-POWELL,
CANCER SURVIVOR AND AUTHOR

Throughout my journey with cancer, one of the most important and powerful lessons I learned is also one of the least tangible. While it's a common saying, "Trust your instincts" is much more easily said than done. However, if you do nothing else offered in this book but trust your instincts, then you will have learned the most important lesson.

That is why this chapter, dedicated to trusting yourself and your instincts, is shared as the first lesson. Like a strong foundation for a house, it's the basis upon which all of the other lessons are built. You know yourself best. Do what *you* think is right.

My instincts have always played a strong role in how I make decisions. When confronted with cancer, I was bombarded with so much emotion, information, and urgency that my instincts were more difficult to identify and access. When I did, however, which I'll explain throughout the book, they never failed me.

In a serious medical situation, it may sound heretical to trust your instincts more than you trust your doctors. After all, medical professionals are highly educated and know more than we do. Decisions are made based on facts and data that we, as regular people, know little about. We have been trained to believe doctors know best. These commonly accepted principles are followed by many patients. Well, medical professionals may know more about medicine, and this is half the game, but they don't know the most about you.

I called upon the power of instinct at the very beginning of my diagnosis, when I had the colonoscopy and later found out I had cancer and would need a colectomy. While the news struck me to my core, I also seemed to know in my heart that everything would be OK. It would have been easier (though none of this is easy!) to just go to the highly recommended local surgeon and move forward with the procedure. If I had not prepared a list of questions and then stepped back to realize I was not completely satisfied with the answers, I may have done just that.

That feeling in my gut of not completely being satisfied with the surgeon's answers nagged at me enough to get a second opinion. It would require more work and more time, both of which I didn't feel I had much of. *Ugh.*

In a recent article in *Psychology Today*, intuition is regarded as a highly sophisticated, pattern-based process. We notice patterns, based on past experiences; store them in long-term memory; and then access them when we see the patterns again in our daily lives. According to the article, the key is determining when to trust it. We are likely to have reliable instincts in areas in which we have extensive experience and practice.

It's estimated that 99 percent of the decisions we make each day, we make without deliberation, meaning based on gut or instinct.[1] Yet when faced with a big decision, and perhaps one with which we have little experience, we tend to fear or ignore our gut. It may be true that we may not know a lot about medicine or the treatment of disease, but there's an awful lot we do know in a general sense about ourselves and others that we can apply to our decision-making process for the best outcome.

Signs and Symbols

The use of signs and symbols to convey meaning and information has been in practice since prehistoric times. In ancient Egypt, symbols seen in dreams were interpreted to help govern, and animal symbolism was often used to emulate qualities humans aspired toward. One of the earliest recorded collections of dream symbols was an Egyptian papyrus text. Today, signs and symbols permeate our culture, though we may no longer see those in government and politics navigating policy and decision-making in quite the same way.

By the time I was diagnosed with cancer, I'd had a lifetime to collect symbols that spoke to me. For example, like many others, I believed that cardinals were a sign from heaven of a loved one. Today I greet cardinals in my yard as "Sarge," my dad, or, when I see a male and female together, as "Nonnie" and "Pap," my grandparents. And as you'll see later in this chapter, the butterfly was a symbol that helped reassure me that I was on the right track, particularly when it came to deciding on the right surgeon for me. The butterfly was a symbol that held true meaning for me and reflected and reassured me that I was on the right track on more than one occasion.

According to the Chopra Center, the world around us is trying to speak to us in our own language of signs and symbols all of the time.[2] The center advocates learning to listen to your intuition and gut instinct by paying close attention to and observing your surroundings for those things that hold meaning for you. With the relentless pace of technology and constant barrage of media, it may be difficult to get quiet enough to see, hear, or even smell symbols that may have meaning for you, but taking the time to think about what symbols hold meaning for you may help you navigate an important part of your cancer journey.

I understand it's easy to go through the day without picking up your head to look around. Life is moving so much more quickly than ever. In fact, my first book, a business book on marketing to women, titled *Too Busy to Shop: Marketing to Multi-Minding Women*, spoke to this trend. Many people, especially women, are already too busy physically and mentally juggling the many dimensions of their to-do lists and lives, never mind stopping to look around for how their environment may be speaking to them. For this reason, I created a game to help teach me to pay more attention in the moment. I picked something to look for in the next few minutes, next few hours, or next day—beige cars, bald men, or anything that worked for me. Gradually this trained me to see outside myself and helped me to tune in to the larger environment, where my values and what was important to me could be reflected back to me. I also developed more appreciation for nature and the world around me.

Susan

I learned that life is much simpler than we make it out to be, and if we insist on being too busy, spread too thin, over-whelmed with this, that, and the other thing, the universe will oblige us in all its knowing glory—until we learn that it's all a big, self-fabricated production, and that the real lesson is in being still and listening, to the lessons, to the birds singing, to the children laughing, to the things that really matter. I learned to watch my grandpa and know that if he—and his mother—made it to nearly one hundred years, that what they were eating and doing must be what we should be doing if a long life is what we're after—so that's what I do. Eat farm to table. Walk every day. Enjoy the moments. Work hard. Take care of the family. Keep friends close.

During my cancer diagnosis and treatment, paying attention to and appreciating the little things in life, especially in nature, helped me. I stayed closer to home. I saw fresh beauty in wildflowers, I took long walks, and I ate simple, homegrown foods from local farms. I had a newfound sense of gratitude for all of the things I'd normally taken for granted.

The butterfly became a meaningful symbol to me because it symbolized transformation, change, hope, and life. But when I first picked the butterfly as my sign, I did so rather arbitrarily; I thought it was rather unusual to see a butterfly and that if I did see one I'd know it was a true sign. I decided that as I encountered butterflies along this journey, it would be a reminder to trust my instincts. I prayed to God, "I don't know why I am on this path, but I am in your hands. Show me a butterfly to let me know it's your path."

Butterflies started to emerge in the most unlikely places.

I mentioned in my personal story that when my husband, mom, and I went for my second opinion, we stopped at the in-hospital Starbucks for coffee. The woman ahead of us in line was a nurse with a surgical cap. The surgical cap had butterflies all over it. My mom pointed it out to me. "I've never seen a surgical cap with butterflies," she said, reflecting on her career as a nurse. After my meeting with the surgeon, I had struggled some on where to have my surgery. Both surgeons were good and qualified, but this surgeon had also given me his cell phone number without blinking. And I'd be lying if I said the butterflies on the surgical cap didn't tip my decision.

When I published my story on *Medium*, titled "Butterflies in my Stomach," I wrote that I had asked God for a sign and looked for butterflies to guide my path. Friends responded by sending me cards and items with butterflies. My dear friend Merry sent a package of all types of butterfly things—magnets, outdoor decorations, and more—to my husband and asked him to secretly place them where I would see them. Each time I saw one, I took it as a reminder to trust my instincts and to remember that I was on the right path. I think I'm still discovering butterflies in my house!

Gratitude

Gratitude is a hot topic these days for good reason. Countless studies have shown that taking the time to think about what you are grateful for and writing it down—making a list or keeping a gratitude journal—can impact your life in several ways, from increased happiness and physical strength to better mental health and improved relationships. Researcher, author, and all-around inspirational role model Brené Brown promotes the power and importance of giving thanks, as do Oprah Winfrey and many others.

When I was diagnosed with cancer and undergoing treatment, I realized just how much I had taken my health and everyday life for granted. Practicing gratitude was an immense help in my treatment and recovery. It wasn't always an easy practice in the beginning, but I became deeply grateful for simple things like being able to put two feet on the ground when I got up and being able to walk up and down steps, and for the nurses who so thoughtfully cared for me. Some of my fellow cancer patients were even more gracious and grateful than I was. One, in particular, shared her gratitude for those who get to ring the end-of-chemo bells.

Mary Kay
....

Sometimes family and friends gather for the bell ringing and celebrating. Hugs are exchanged. Pictures are taken. Smiles are wide! In 2014, I was blessed with cancer for the second time in my life. The official medical diagnosis was Stage IV metastatic breast cancer. On various occasions while sitting in the oncologist's office waiting for my treatment, I have heard the "survival bell." The person who was privileged to ring the survival bell would then walk through the waiting area to additional claps and shouts of support. I have smiled, clapped, and whispered prayers for them. All the time knowing I will never ring the bell. Never will I be considered cancer-free. My treatments will never be complete. The survival bell, I believe, rings for all touched by cancer. The bell rings for those with cancer as well as those that are now cancer-free. It rings for caregivers and staff, for family and friends. The bell is a symbol; you get to choose what the bell means. When the bell rings, it makes me smile. I am sincerely happy for the bell ringer. I am happy to be alive. I am happy to be a survivor. The bell for me means "Believe Everyone Loves Life." For as long as the Lord permits, I will live, grow, learn, and prosper with my cancer diagnosis. This is my personal opportunity to discover and cherish all the doctors, nurses, aides, and experiences that will be a part of my cancer journey. I am blessed.

Author's note: Sadly, in 2020, the remarkable Miss Mary Kay Plank passed away after a long and blessed life living with cancer.

I developed a twenty-to-thirty-minute meditation practice that helped me learn to trust my instincts, pay more attention to the world around me, and cultivate gratitude. This practice may also work for you. To start, I found a quiet place in the house to sit—usually the lounger in my bedroom. Once seated, I closed my eyes and focused on my breathing, taking long, deep breaths. When my breathing became deep and even, I made a mental gratitude list that I shared with God of all of the things for which I was grateful. Then I shared any concerns I had about my experiences or life and asked for guidance. Clearing my mind, learning to listen, and focusing my energy on my body played a significant role in my healing. Often, in the hours after these sessions, I'd have fresh insights to problems. This practice is something I try to do now, even if just for a few minutes.

While much easier, admittedly, when you are healthy, my pattern of gratitude continues today. Every day I try to be cognizant of each wonderful part of my life and give thanks in my mind and through a nightly practice of gratitude journaling.

Taking Action on Learning to Trust Your Instincts

▶ Find Quiet Time and Still Your Mind

When faced with an anxiety-laden situation, many of us seek answers online or from doctors, friends, and anyone who has an opinion. While it requires some discipline, I found twenty minutes of quiet time a day more helpful than all the noise. In that quiet time, I focused on what I really wanted—to be healthy—and deep breathing.

▶ Pick Your "Sign"

As you quiet your mind, think about signs that would be meaningful but not all that common. Land on a sign and ask God, or the Universe, or whatever energy you may believe in, to show you your sign when needed. When you see it, let it remind you not to waffle and to believe in your gut. You will be amazed at how your signs will appear to guide your path.

▶ *Look Around and Pay Attention*
Butterflies became a sign that I decided to pay attention to, and they started appearing in the most unlikely of places, as I have explained earlier in this chapter. The simple and beautiful things in nature and in life were also things I started to pay attention to—the colors of sunset, the delicious taste of a strong cup of coffee in the morning, singing birds, the amazing structure of a gorgeous flower bloom.

▶ *Give Thanks*
What am I grateful for today? It ranges from the physical to the emotional and everything in between: perfect health, a full house, a loving husband, great kids, a wonderful family, meaningful work, great clients, abundance, and my cats are included every day. My gratitude somehow seems to reinforce my instincts and let me focus on what is most important.

Don't let the seeming simplicity of the ways to learn to trust your instincts fool you. They are simple, but they are not always easy. They require a firm decision to activate and discipline to do. But if you do, you will be amazed at how they work, as I was. Trust your instincts. Trust yourself and how you feel, even if someone like a doctor has more pure medical knowledge.

In summary, here are four things you can do to take action on trusting your instincts:

1. Find quiet time and still your mind.
2. Pick your sign, and look for it each and every day.
3. Look around, especially at nature, and pay attention to small details and gestures that may be meaningful and lift your spirits.
4. Write down three things you are grateful for every day.

CHAPTER 3:

Do Your Research

It's about focusing on the fight, not the fright.
—ROBIN ROBERTS, CANCER SURVIVOR
AND TELEVISION HOST

Doctors have lost their edge as the most-trusted source of medical information to the Internet. Historically, a person had to wait for an appointment or a callback from a doctor to find out anything about his or her medical condition. Patients took the doctors' word as gospel, not questioning their opinion and without other resources to educate them on their conditions or guide them in their treatments. While this has not been true in my adult lifetime, I do remember these dynamics when my grandparents needed treatment for health problems, and several cancer-treatment patients I have encountered have depended on doctors as their main source of information and knowledge.

Many people, including doctors, have suggested, "Don't google your sickness." But how else can you best advocate for yourself if you haven't done your research, your homework? How will you know what questions to ask? How will you know what to expect? How will you know how to best prepare yourself? To me, forewarned is to be forearmed. Others may subscribe to the idea that ignorance is bliss, but I believe that knowledge is power, and it has always served me better than ignorance.

Many cancer patients seem to see their doctors as the font of all knowledge. Doctors are certainly knowledgeable, though your doctor is one expert in a world and field of many.

Thankfully, the trend of implicitly trusting a health condition to one expert is changing. According to a recent study by the Pew Internet & American Life Project, the number of people turning to the Internet to search for a diverse range of health-related subjects continues to grow. "In all, 80 percent of Internet users, or about 93 million Americans, have searched for a health-related topic online. That's up from 62 percent of Internet users who went online for health topics in 2001."[1] Further, looking up information on a specific disease or medical problem tops the list (63 percent) of searches. That's a lot of homework being done on a platform that doctors widely regard as the place *not* to go.

Online Research

While sometimes a scary place to roam, the Internet was helpful to me because I knew so little about colon cancer. I found it helpful to scan sites ranging from the American Cancer Society to WebMD. The information was reputable and thorough and gave me my footing, though it was daunting to suddenly be thrown into the online world of cancer. There was as much scary information as there was helpful information.

The colectomy surgery appeared to be the most common and proven surgery at my stage, and I took comfort in knowing this course of action was standard. Perhaps more significant was what I found through my research on chemotherapy treatment. I found out that certain doctors are used to working with certain drugs and treating a certain type of cancer patient, and that the chemo regimen was not very personalized but rather was based on clinical trials. When I later began experiencing serious side effects during my chemo treatment, I couldn't help but think my chemo regimen didn't fit me.

Not wanting to precondition my mind to expect certain side effects, I tried not to look at the side effects of the chemo drugs during my research. Chemo side effects can be worse than the chemo treatment itself. However, when my side effects became so debilitatingly toxic, I broke down and explored message boards and tried to discern just how bad my side effects were, relatively speaking. I learned that my side effects were extremely bad, compared to most other patients. This knowledge gave me the reinforcement and support I needed to speak up.

Ask a Nurse

Professional resources are another effective avenue of research. Almost everyone knows a nurse or has a friend or family member who does. Nurses are smart, accessible, and helpful. They see a wide range of conditions and can be knowledgeable and compassionate resources. In a 2019 Gallup poll, nursing ranked as the most trusted profession for the twentieth year in a row.[2]

When looking for honest yet compassionate input while doing my homework, nurses were at the top of my list. Fortunately for me, my family has always been blessed with an in-house nurse, my mom, who was an operating room nurse for many years. Her medical knowledge was invaluable to me, and she attended many doctor's appointments with me to give me a second opinion.

She has seen it all, and if she couldn't render a full opinion, she knew someone who could. Her knowledge and contacts, as well as her compassion, were incredibly helpful to me.

My mom put me in touch with another specialty nurse, a head nurse anesthetist, who took time to explain the complex topic of anesthesia as well as my options and did so in a way that provided great comfort. This nurse anesthetist spoke with medical terms but also translated them into language that I could understand, like she was talking to someone in her family—with respect, care, and relevant knowledge.

Lisa

....

When I was diagnosed with Stage I uterine cancer, one of the best pieces of advice came from a retired and candid nurse named Hazel who lived across the street from me. I told Hazel I wanted to keep my ovaries if they were in good health. "What they don't tell you when you get a radical hysterectomy is all your parts fall out your vagina and you may have to get a mesh implant," Hazel said. Hazel's candid comment and advice made me fight even harder to keep my ovaries. My doctor agreed to leave them in if they looked healthy . . . and eventually did so. By keeping my ovaries, I still enjoy their protective health benefits to my bones and heart and avoided the very real possibility of further complications and surgeries.

When I would later undergo chemo, the oncology nurses were fonts of knowledge on the clinical side and were well-versed in practical knowledge, like which doctors consistently ran late. The oncology nurses became a lifeline for me, literally and figuratively, and I owe them a debt of gratitude. If you are being treated by an oncology nurse, be especially kind to them.

Anesthesia

Anesthesia was a key concern for me, and I spent a great deal of time researching this area. It's funny: most people seem to accept anesthesia as an unquestioned part of surgery. In talking with a nurse who I encountered in a recent, routine colonoscopy, he noted that I was the only person he's ever heard ask about anesthesia, and he didn't understand why. When you think about it, anesthesia is a powerful drug, and your body will have to adapt and react, adding another layer to recovery. Perhaps what you don't know you don't worry about, but, as I've said, I'm a "knowledge is power" person.

As I mentioned above, one nurse anesthetist was particularly helpful in helping me think through the standards of care and my options. In addition, the daily news provided a great deal of information about one class of drugs that is used in both anesthesia and common postoperative pain management—opioids.

Opioids

You likely know there is a serious opioid epidemic in our country. Sadly, every day you read news about how opioids are being overprescribed, are illegally transported into our country, or are the cause of death of someone. In fact, 130 deaths per day are attributed to opioids in just the US. These same drugs are used as a standard of care to treat patients for pain from surgeries like a colectomy or hysterectomy.

Back in the 1990s, pharmaceutical companies reassured the medical community that patients would not become addicted to opioid pain relievers, and healthcare providers began to prescribe them at greater rates. According to the United States Department of Health and Human Services, "Increased prescription of opioid medications led to widespread misuse of both prescription and non-prescription opioids before it became clear that these medications could indeed be highly addictive."[3] Now we know that addiction can happen in just five days. In 2017, the United States Department of Health and Human Services declared opioids a public health emergency. Yet opioids are being used and offered to patients every day.

A dear friend of mine who had recently undergone a double mastectomy cautioned me to ask about opioid use in my surgeries. She had discovered that opioids were used as a routine part of her care. Out of concern for her sensitive system and the potential addictive properties of opioids, she worked with her medical team to avoid them.

Given her advice, I did the same. Prior to having my colonoscopy, colectomy, and port surgery (the annoying device inserted into my chest wall to enable infusion therapy to bypass my veins), I called ahead of time and asked to speak to the anesthesiologist. My body's system is very sensitive, and I notice the effects of things as harmless as vitamins, so I was curious and cautious about the use of anesthesia.

As it turned out, fentanyl, a synthetic opioid, is commonly used in surgery. While I questioned each use and made it clear that I did not want opioids used, there were few options for surgical pain management. While addiction does not usually occur from surgical use, I didn't want these substances in my body, but I found through my research that I had no choice.

Where I did have a choice, however, was after my colectomy surgery. I elected to be part of a fast recovery protocol that eliminated the usually prescribed opioids and called only for the use of Tylenol. For me, it worked just fine. Before I was released from the hospital, I was offered a prescription for an opioid painkiller in case I needed it. I didn't need it or want it, so I turned it down.

Clearly, the opportunity is present, post-surgery, for many people to gain access to opioids even if they don't want or need them. It's a dangerous practice and one I decided to take control of by not accepting the prescription, even when offered opioids a year after my surgery. "You are not the norm," the nurse said, which still surprised me. "Many people are fearful of pain."

In further research I found he was right. The National Institutes of Health surveyed patients and found that "concerns regarding persistent opioid use after surgery include misuse, abuse, addiction, and diversion. . . . The potential for misuse and diversion is highlighted by research reporting that the majority of patients keep their unused opioids rather than disposing of them after surgery."[4]

Though I'm not known for high pain tolerance, Tylenol worked just fine for me. Everyone is different, and you need to do what you need to do if pain is debilitating. But using opioids can present a bigger, more painful situation in many ways in the longer term, so consider wisely.

Nutrition

While many facets of surgery and cancer treatment are routinely covered during doctors' visits and with informational packets, important topics like nutrition and holistic treatments, referred to as "integrative medicine," are rarely covered in discussions and are not covered by insurance. I found this truth shocking. Practicing good nutrition is one of the most important things you can do to help with healing, and yet it's apparently not part of a medical approach, and few doctors want to or are knowledgeable enough about it to discuss the topic.

Why isn't nutrition an integral part of medicine? I wish I had a definitive answer. Nutrition is not a major part of medical school or training. That's because our medical system revolves around drugs, which are the basis of clinical trials and considered to be the gold standard in determining effective treatment and care. In my opinion, it comes back to money. Foods and nutritional supplements can't be patented and aren't drivers of big money, so the research to determine their medical effectiveness pales in comparison to drug research, which can result in big money to pharmaceutical companies.

During my many years in marketing, I have worked with dozens of clients in the food and wellness arenas—major brands we all know and love—so I have been exposed to nutrition research of many kinds. A healthful eater by nature and choice, I had routinely taken note of nutrition research and adapted my diet accordingly.

Nutrition research was not foreign to me, though researching how to combat the side effects of chemo was a surprising new addition. Limiting sugar and upping my intake of cruciferous vegetables, like kale and broccoli, were things I incorporated. At the same time, I learned that taking some of the supplements that I normally used and that seemed more needed than ever could actually decrease the effectiveness of the chemo, like antioxidants, vitamin C, vitamin E, and beta-carotene. In addition to online searches that yielded massive amounts of findings, I also made an appointment with an integrative medicine specialist—which I ended up feeling particularly thankful for, because the nutritionist in the chemo infusion center was right out of the 1950s in her approach to nutrition. (Her go-to suggestions for the extreme side effects of chemo were drinking Ensure and slathering butter on everything.)

The specialist recommended a variety of natural supplements that could be used in place of or in addition to pharmaceuticals to reduce the impact of chemo. I ended up using several of the recommended supplements and found them helpful, and certainly better than more drugs. For example, I experienced the very common post-chemo nausea. The normal course of action is another prescription drug to combat nausea. While I didn't want to use another drug to combat the side effects of the chemo drug, I tried it, but I didn't get relief. A ginger supplement, recommended by the integrative medicine specialist, was more effective for me in fighting nausea. In fact, I ended up sharing my "integrative medicine" solutions with several patients in the chemo infusion center because they were experiencing similar issues. Some of the supplements, like turmeric, I continue to take today.

I am truly a believer in healing cancer through nutrition. I am a believer that food is medicine. But you'll find that healing food and nutrition seemed to be totally outside the realm of helping cancer patients heal. Do your research to find out how you can improve your healing process through food and nutritional supplementation.

Ovie

In 2005, there wasn't much information on the Internet in regards to nutrition during cancer treatments. My husband, who was a chiropractor and finishing his master's in clinical nutrition at the time, was a huge help. He reached out to professors that had taught his classes for help, and we started on nutrients to boost the immune system, such as superfood shakes, high doses of vitamin C and Carnivora, and limited sugar and dairy. Fast-forward fifteen years, and I do so much more for prevention of cancer, especially working with a functional doctor who can monitor my levels of CA 27-29 (tumor marker) and vitamin D and NK cells, along with detoxing all the toxins out of my body, through PEMF (pulse electromagnetic frequency), ionic foot baths, far-infrared saunas, hair analysis (heavy metals), hormonal testing, and also seeing a biological dentist for removal of mercury fillings as well as juicing.

The Chemo "Holiday," or Break

Chemotherapy is an ugly, painful course of treatment, but it's the accepted standard of care for treating some stages of cancer. According to the Centers for Disease Control and Prevention, each year about six hundred and fifty thousand cancer patients receive chemotherapy in an outpatient oncology clinic in the United States.[5]

About a month into my three-month chemo regimen, the side effects from the chemo drugs became unbearable. I was unable to eat much or smell food. I became nauseous and plagued with horrible digestive pain. I had blisters the size of dimes on my toes and round-the-clock diarrhea. This physical depletion also wreaked havoc on my mind.

Because I was no longer able to withstand the chemo, my oncologist recommended a chemo break. This break, or time off (sometimes referred to as a "chemo holiday," ha!), is needed to rebuild the body's tolerance to the drug.

Though chemo is well-documented, one area where I was surprised to come up blank in my research was "chemo breaks." Through my research and in talking with others, I realized that this happens much more often than is acknowledged by doctors or in clinical trial documentation. My research also revealed that there was no "science" to a chemo break, how long it should be, and if the break impacts the outcome of the course of treatment. My oncologist said that breaks have not been well studied and that it's where the "art versus the science" of medicine takes over. The science was telling me to power through, but my body was telling me that I might not survive if I did.

Google works magic for many things, but definitive information on chemo breaks is like searching for a needle in a haystack. Through many online searches, I found many people talking about the breaks, especially on message boards, but I could not find any definitive information. The message boards showed that quite a few people needed to take breaks and that some never resumed treatment because of the side effects. Given the prevalence of needed breaks, to me this showed there is a gap in the medical research in this area that desperately needs to be filled. It also reinforced the reality that treatment isn't formulated for the individual.

What were the implications of treatment success on an amended schedule? No one knew. The clinical trials didn't account for any treatment suspension or lower doses over more time. I could not find a shred of research that took an amended treatment schedule into consideration, though in reality many patients needed an amended regimen.

Financial Obligations

When you are diagnosed with cancer and have to undergo months, or years, of intense medical treatment, it comes at a cost, physically, mentally, and literally. While it may be something you'd rather ignore, medical financial obligations are an important area to research and educate yourself about.

Though I was always one to be on top of my finances, I simply didn't even think of financial consequences when I was diagnosed. With good health insurance, I just moved forward with the course of care that my physicians and I came to agree on. Never, not once, were costs mentioned or shown or did I proactively ask.

Crazy, right? We know what we'll pay when we purchase anything else in life, but with healthcare, costs are a mystery. With cancer, it's an expensive mystery. About a month after my first procedure, I started receiving insurance statements. The numbers were staggering, but my insurance covered most of it.

As time went on, the statements and bills kept coming. I started to budget at least $500 a month, in addition to the monthly insurance premium, to cover my medical expenses. Within a few months, I had reached my personal maximum deductible of over $5,000.

Not only were the bills staggering in terms of amounts, but there were so many of them! At one point, I mistakenly but repeatedly threw away invoices from one particular provider. This was normally something I'd never do, and I struggled to keep track. This particular provider sent my account to a collections agency, which sent me sixty-seven separate bills, many for less than $1.

Based on my research, the average cost to treat cancer runs around $150,000, so my case was average. All told, my bills amounted to close to $150,000. I also maxed out my personal deductible for two years, so I ended up spending over $10,000 in additional healthcare expenses.

My dear friend, Andrea, was much better prepared than I was. She shares some sage advice, below.

Andrea

I was very fortunate to receive treatment at a comprehensive cancer center. Once my standard of care was decided, I met with a financial manager at the center, who took my insurance card and then told me that in a few days she'd have an idea of what my full financial obligations would be for my treatment, including having my medical port inserted. I returned a week later, and the first thing she said to me was, "You have very good insurance." She then listed all of the items that would be covered, and those that would require a co-payment. She said that of my total bill—$350,000—I would be responsible for about $7,000. She also told me that every month or so, I'd get a huge bill of about $30,000. I was to disregard it, put it in a drawer, and wait until the insurance company resolved my insurance. She was right. Every few weeks I'd get a bill for an enormous amount of money. The bill always arrived on Friday, just after I returned from my weekly treatment, and always after 5 p.m. when I could no longer reach anyone at the insurance company. It always stated that I owed the amount immediately—it made me worry, but not half as much as I would have if I had not met with the financial manager. Knowing upfront what my financial obligations were was extremely helpful and reduced a lot of my stress over finances. My advice is to work with your hospital's financial team to understand obligations before treatment. Work with them, or a patient advocate, who can work with your insurance company to outline your financial plan.

Though so many questions in medicine remain, doing diligent home-work can help create a sense that knowledge is power and can help you take back control of your health. Learning more from your doctor, nurses, trusted friends, and family; from research conducted on your condition or treatment; and, yes, from Google will help you become better prepared. Though you may not be eager to learn about anesthesia and opioids, that learning will help you navigate your situation and feel more in control.

Taking Action on Doing Your Research

▶ *Google It*

Contrary to what most doctors say about not googling a sickness or health problem, I say Google it. Do, however, look to reputable sources for your information. Even though I'm in the marketing business, I skip any of the top search results that are ads and then look for WebMD, the Cleveland Clinic, and the American Cancer Society.

▶ *Read the Clinical Trials*

Look for clinical trials that were done and white papers written for any drugs or therapies that are recommended for you. These documents are dense and complicated, but you will be surprised how quickly you learn and understand medical terms when they relate directly to you or someone you love. Pay special attention to the demographics in the study—the gender and age of those enrolled in the trial—to see if they reflect your age and gender. If not, be aware that how you react to the course of treatment may differ from those in the study.

▶ *Talk to Others*

Even though it seems that medicine is an advanced science with studies to underpin so many health challenges, there are gaps in science and knowledge. Talking with other people who have been in similar situations may help you fill in those gaps, as will trusting your instincts with what you think is the best course of action for you.

▶ *Ask a Nurse*

Reach out to your favorite nurse—almost everyone knows one. They are knowledgeable, compassionate, and helpful. Ask your favorite nurse if he or she can refer you to someone else who is an expert in your area of questioning. Nurses are very connected in the medical community.

▶ *Keep Abreast of Relevant News*

Keep track of what's happening in the news with opioids. Explore your options with online research before you have a doctor's appointment. Ask the doctor about the standards of care related to drugs used. Insist on talking to the anesthesiologist before you go in for surgery or treatment, and create a plan that suits you.

▶ *Seek Out Alternative Therapies*

Explore integrative medicine options in your community, and make an appointment to talk with someone about the specifics of your situation. I found the nonpharmaceutical approach to be much more in line with my thinking and my body. The appointment and the supplements are very likely not covered by insurance, which should change, but I found them worth the investment.

▶ *Understand Financial Obligations*

Actively seek out financial information and help. Understand, upfront, what your insurance will cover and what your personal financial responsibility will be. Know that the invoices will be daunting and that you don't need to deal with them immediately. Let the provider and the insurance company work out their payments, and, in the meantime, try not to worry or let the numbers upset you.

In summary, here are seven things you can do to take action on doing your research:

1. Google any condition or term you want to understand.
2. Read the clinical trials, and make note of whether the participating patients reflect your age and stage of cancer.
3. Talk to others with similar circumstances.
4. Ask a nurse for advice.
5. Keep abreast of relevant news.
6. Seek out alternative therapies, such as nutrition.
7. Understand your financial obligations.

CHAPTER 4:

Prepare to Speak Up

The only person I know who can save you is you. That was going to be the thing that informed the rest of my life.
—SHERYL CROW, CANCER SURVIVOR
AND SINGER

From politics and parenting to celebrities and causes, speaking out and speaking up seem to be commonplace in our world. There is no shortage of opinions shared on even the toughest of subjects, except, it seems, when it comes to our own health advocacy. What I discovered, however, is what I am calling the self-advocacy triple whammy: a dangerous combination of human nature, being a woman, and having cancer.

A recent article in *Forbes* noted that "speaking up powerfully for oneself is one of the most universal challenges human beings face today." While many people speak out about many things, speaking up for yourself is not nearly as common. The article went on to note that "it's particularly difficult for women the world over, given how our society and culture trains both men and women to think and behave, and shapes how we all perceive assertiveness."[1]

Having spent decades in the marketing industry working with powerful women and men, I have seen the tendency firsthand for women to advocate strongly for others but neglect to speak up for themselves. Whether it's a result of politeness or uncertainty, many women tend to not speak up, or not speak up loudly enough.

Now translate those dynamics to a healthcare setting, and a serious one at that. Patients receive all kinds of information about their courses of treatment. I received a thick binder full of information (yes—a good old-fashioned three-ring white binder right out of the 1980s) when I had my first chemo appointment. There are pages and pages of details just on the drugs, full of complex explanations and words.

Despite the deluge of information, a study on patient self-advocacy in *Psychology Today* reports that "less than half [of patients] report being knowledgeable about their treatment options, and a significant proportion reported not having enough knowledge or support to fully engage in treatment decisions." I'm not surprised. Further, "Over half felt significantly unprepared to discuss treatment options with their doctor. . . . It is not uncommon for patients not to report all of their symptoms and side-effects from treatment to the health care team."[2]

Speaking up is important, critically important, and, in fact, encouraging patients to speak up about problems that occur during hospitalizations can improve patient experience and safety, research indicates. I was often frustrated that I was the only one who knew fully what my story and situation was. But patients are uniquely qualified to raise concerns about care because they are often the only one present for the full spectrum of care. Most patients do not raise concerns or file formal complaints, according to research, with hesitancy to speak up linked to several factors, such as an expectation that complaining will not make a difference.

A study published in the *Journal of Clinical Oncology* notes that "cancer treatments are complex, involving multiple clinicians, toxic therapies, and uncertain outcomes. . . . Consequently, patients are vulnerable when breakdowns in care occur." Further, "Cancer patients who believe they experienced a preventable, harmful event during their cancer diagnosis or care often do not formally report their concerns. Systems are needed to encourage patients to report such events and to help physicians and health care systems respond effectively."[3]

These findings suggest that problematic events experienced by patients in cancer care may be relatively common and physically and emotionally harmful, and that they often are not formally reported. As healthcare institutions strive to develop patient-centered cultures of care, additional consideration should be given to how improved communication with patients could prevent problems in care and could facilitate effective responses.

Why Don't Patients Speak Up?

A study recently published in *BMJ Journals* explored the important question of why patients don't speak up. Patients frequently experience problems in care during hospitalization, and many do not feel comfortable speaking up. According to a study of 10,212 patients who provided valid responses, 4,958 (48.6 percent) indicated they had experienced a problem during hospitalization. Of these, 1,514 (30.5 percent) did not always feel comfortable speaking up.

Predictors of having a problem during hospitalization included age, health status, and education level.[4] The study went on to conclude that "creating conditions for patients to be comfortable speaking up may result in service recovery opportunities and improved patient experience."

Though I hadn't previously heard of a program called Speak Up, as I was writing this book, my research brought it to my attention, and I thought it was worth sharing. The Joint Commission accredits and certifies nearly twenty-one thousand healthcare organizations and programs in the United States. Since 2002, The Joint Commission has helped the public play an active role in their care by providing free, downloadable education materials through the Speak Up program. Recently relaunched in May 2018, the revamped Speak Up program is based on national market research conducted in 2017. A focus group of patients and their family caregivers was tapped to provide feedback on the program.

The program emphasizes that everyone has a role in making healthcare safe––physicians, nurses, healthcare workers, and, guess who, You! As the patient, you play a critical role in how you receive care. You must be active, informed, and vocal. In short, you must speak up.

Anna

....

When I learned that technicians were going to tattoo dots on my breast and chest to help them guide the radiation beams during my six weeks of treatments, I felt an instant rebellion build up inside of me. Not because I was afraid of pain or because I had anything in particular against tattoos but because as far as I was concerned, the breast cancer was a one-time deal, and when the treatments were over, I planned on forgetting all about it. I didn't want to be reminded of the ordeal for the rest of my life every time I looked in the mirror. I understood why they would do it, but I also understood that I had the right to question any procedure. As I lay on the table while technicians were taking measurements of my chest and clavicle area and making marks for the tattoos with what appeared to be a magic marker, I suddenly blurted out, "I don't want the tattoos!" My unexpected declaration was followed by a prolonged silence. I could feel my heartbeat rise in anticipation. Finally, the silence was broken by one of the technicians explaining that they needed the markings to stay put throughout the treatments. Knowing that it's not easy to wash off magic marker from skin, I continued my plight. "I can touch them up with the marker every day so they won't fade." After another period of silence, they relented, making me promise to make sure that the markings remained visible. I breathed a sigh of relief, confirming my belief that if you feel strongly about something or something doesn't feel right, you should never be afraid to speak up.

One month into my chemo regimen, I was in dire straits due to side effects, and I found it hard to speak up. Self-doubt about my condition, a significant loss of energy, not getting much of a reaction from the medical team, and not wanting to be a pain in someone's ass all contributed to my reticence. But when I got to the point when my physical and mental ability to withstand treatment was fading, I had to find the strength to save myself. It's crazy that I had to get to such a breaking point before pressing harder to get a response from my doctor.

Don't let yourself get to this point. If things don't seem right to you, then they aren't. Speak up for yourself, even if you feel like you are being a pain. Find the strength to speak up for yourself before you lose your strength altogether.

Taking Action on Preparing to Speak Up

▶ *Own Your Advocacy*

As a cancer patient, you will be weakened, scared, and in unfamiliar territory. Don't let these things deter you from the truth that you are your own best advocate. No one knows what you know about what you are feeling and going through like you do. Do for yourself what you would do for your child—ask questions, get answers, press on if needed, and don't ever feel bad about owning your advocacy.

▶ *Take Notes*

One of the easiest and most effective ways I was able to advocate for myself was by keeping a running notebook of everything that happened to me—doctors' visits, questions, symptoms, medications—anything related to my healthcare. My notebook became my nonelectronic medical record and proved to be more reliable than the electronic healthcare records kept by the doctors. I always had my notes, dates, and questions in one place and could more easily reference symptoms and procedures by date than could the medical team.

With some of my treatment, I was dealing with cooperating but different healthcare systems. And guess what, their electronic records didn't talk to each other, so my notebook served as a resource to both myself and the medical teams. While I hope you never need to create a "calendar of pain and suffering," the calendar itself was a valuable tool that you might want to incorporate into your notebook.

▶ *Bring the Same Person with You to Critical Appointments*

My husband and often my mom, the nurse, accompanied me on the most important doctors' appointments and treatments, especially when I was in an emotional or weakened state. They listened and asked questions, too. Having them in the room provided comfort to me, and they served as an extra set of ears and eyes. Though I was sometimes too numb to ask anything other than the questions I had prepared in my notebook, my husband and mom listened with fresher minds and were helpful in being more responsive and reactive in the moment as well as serving as sounding boards after an appointment.

▶ *Access Online Resources*

There are various online resources that can help prepare you to advocate for yourself, like the educational materials from The Joint Commission's Speak Up. Just understanding how common not speaking up is and how hard it is to do gave me a degree of comfort and reassurance. When you read the statistics and realize that speaking up improves outcomes, then it should become as routine as taking prescribed medication.

In summary, here are five things you can do to take action to prepare to speak up:

1. Be prepared to be your own best advocate.
2. Take notes throughout your cancer journey, especially before and during appointments.
3. Bring the same person with you to critical appointments.
4. Access online resources.
5. Muster the strength to speak up for yourself.

CHAPTER 5:

Know Your Medical History

Cancer woke me up to my health, and I feel like
I've been given a second chance.
—LORRAINE HUTCHINSON, CANCER SURVIVOR
AND DEPUTY FIRE CHIEF

They say that history repeats itself. When it comes to your medical history and any serious illness, you'll repeat yourself again and again and again (and again and again) as each medical provider—doctor, nurse, resident—needs to hear the details of your condition. Of course, you want each medical provider to know what's going on and have the latest details. The more you know—and the more you keep track of your medical history—the better prepared you'll be to navigate cancer treatment or treatment of any complex or chronic health issues.

The repetition can be aggravating. I considered videotaping my story on my phone so I could just push "play." At several points I even refused to repeat my story to residents because I didn't want to waste my time and become irritated by having to repeat the same thing to the doctor a few minutes later. This approach was not well-received.

When you are diagnosed with cancer, your medical history builds on an almost-daily basis, with tests, treatments, reactions, medications, and procedures that have you in a doctor's office or treatment facility more frequently than ever before. It's easy to lose track and assume that someone, somewhere in the medical system has an accurate and up-to-date accounting of your history and your records. In fact, it's not an unrealistic expectation. It's just not what happens.

With so much talk in the news about electronic medical records, I assumed that the reality of medical care matched the hype of the ease of electronic records. It only makes sense that since five-year-olds now effectively communicate electronically that highly educated and trained medical professionals and institutions could do the same. But *au contraire, mon frere*. Even within cooperating medical institutions, medical records are not as easily available as one would think.

Not having quick access to my medical records or needing to have records available at multiple treatment facilities revealed the flaws in the system to me. These inefficiencies led to delays and high levels of frustration for me as a patient. In talking with other cancer patients, many still just trust in the medical institutions to take responsibility for their medical history and records and accept delays as part of medical care. I did not and still do not.

Many people do not know nearly as much as they should about their medical records, including how to access and use them. It's confusing and frustrating to be in charge of your medical records, to be sure, but it's very useful when being treated for cancer.

HIPAA

Most of us who have extensive experience with the healthcare system have been asked to sign a HIPAA form prior to getting treatment. HIPAA protects our medical information and restricts access to only those who have our (patient) approval. The flip side to that policy is that access to your health records is a patient right protected under HIPAA, which is a law.

Under the Health Insurance Portability and Accountability Act of 1996, patients have a right to get some or all of their medical records upon request.[1] Medical institutions, including hospitals, physician practices, pharmacies, and health insurers, are required to make records information available within thirty days at a reasonable cost and in the format that the patient requests.

Though HIPAA has been around for quite a while, according to a study published in the *Journal of AHIMA* (the American Health Information Management Association), 27 percent of patients don't know they have a HIPAA-protected right to have a copy of any kind of their medical records, and 41 percent say they have never even seen their own health information. Yikes! Yet, eight in ten people who view their medical records consider that information useful.[2] According to the GetMyHealthData initiative, 78 percent of people who get copies of their health records have better communication with their doctors.

Keep Records

In my experience, personally kept, old-school, hard-copy records were the holy grail. For example, early on in my diagnosis, when I had a CT for my colon that included my chest, the scan showed something in my left breast. In addition to dealing with colon cancer, I now had to explore the possibility of breast cancer. An emergency diagnostic mammogram was in order.

Over the prior ten years, I'd had mammograms at the same hospital. When I tried to schedule the emergency diagnostic mammogram, this same hospital could not take me for ten days. Not kidding, *ten* days. Ten days is ten lifetimes when you are wrestling with cancer, so I called another hospital to see if they could take me sooner.

Yes. They could take me sooner, thank God, in three days. I called my past provider, got copies of all my films and past mammogram results—all of which I had an immediate right to—and hand-delivered them to the new mammogram provider. I had an appointment within three days.

While I wish it had been easier and faster, especially given the stress I was under, I learned a lesson in surviving the healthcare system.

Thankfully, the diagnostic mammogram came back clear.

The diagnostic mammogram process was what initially taught me to be a steward of my own medical records. Taking matters into my own hands—and you must take matters into yours—I discovered that any patient can go to a hospital's records department and get copies of his or her own records. I called in advance to request my years of mammogram films, told them I'd be there the next day to get them, marched myself over to the mammogram facility, and got copies of those records. With records in hand, the other facility would see me. Once they examined my films, I took them back and kept them in my files.

This exercise was one I began to repeat with each procedure and test. It's extra work, but it's very well worth it. I collected copies of each record, result, film, or other documentation and kept it in my healthcare journal. Anytime I was talking with a doctor or nurse, I had the information at my fingertips before they did. And it didn't matter if I was being treated at facilities in different hospital systems, which I was. The reports and test results were always accessible via my personal records.

Keeping the records in my own possession was as helpful to me as it was to the medical professionals. In the throes of treatment, there are so many medical details to consider, and your memory fades a bit under the deluge of data and stress. I ended up referring to my records on an almost-daily basis and took great comfort in knowing I had the details within my control. Maybe I'm just Type A (not maybe . . . I *know* I'm Type A), but having control over something within cancer treatment is also a major coup.

Ovie

....

I learned early on to look at what surgery, chemo, and radiation was going to do for me instead of to me, as we know the treatments are worse than the disease itself. Remember, your treatment has a beginning and an ending, and you want the outcome to be cancer-free. You're in charge of your treatment plan. Research your cancer. Do you have a family history? What is the possible cause of this cancer? Get copies of every test, blood work, and doctors' notes to keep in a file. Research your doctors, make sure you feel comfortable with them, and trust your feelings. If it doesn't feel right, it's not!

The number of records grew and grew, so I had to shift from a notebook to a file folder to an expandable file folder. That folder was lugged to each and every appointment. I still use that folder and collect records from my follow-up checkups, referred to as "surveillance." Most cancer patients will have follow-up appointments to monitor their condition for five years after treatment.

At my one-year checkup, they did not have the record from my colonoscopy, which was done at a different but cooperating medical facility. Given I had colon cancer, having the results of a colonoscopy would be one of the most important records to have. They didn't. I did.

Prior to that oncologist appointment, a CT scan and blood work were required. For these tests, I let the technician know that I wanted the results as soon as they were available, which was usually within twenty-four to forty-eight hours. Then I went to the medical records department at the hospital and picked up and read the results myself. With cancer, waiting in uncertainty can cause major stress. This way, I retained my own records and had a heads-up on the results, so I didn't have to wait days before meeting with a doctor to share the information.

Thank God, all results were normal. If they hadn't been, I would have called the doctor and asked for a phone consultation as soon as possible in order to get a read on what was happening so I wouldn't have to wait days worrying.

Perhaps this head-on, direct approach is not for everyone. For many, reading test results on their own may be confusing, though you can learn enough as a patient to decipher much prior to talking with your doctor. Even if you don't want to read your own results, maintaining your own copies of your medical records will absolutely help you to be prepared, reduce wait times, and fill the gaps in the medical-records situations that you will undoubtedly find.

Taking Action on Knowing Your Medical History

▶ HIPAA

While we gloss over so much of the overly complicated medical forms that we sign, it's worth knowing and understanding how HIPAA protects you and your rights to your records. All you have to do is act on those rights and ask for your records and obtain them.

▶ Start a File

As soon as you are diagnosed with cancer, you will be deluged with information, mostly hard-copy printouts, pamphlets, and other information that you'll need to read and refer back to. Find yourself a large, sturdy folder, and file your important information in one place for easy reference.

▶ *Become Your Own Record-Keeper*
With so much on your mind, it's easier to leave the record- and file-keeping to the professionals. After all, they have an electronic record system and know what they are doing, right? In my experience, you cannot expect speed and accuracy if you depend on doctor's offices to manage your records. You can speed up the process of knowing your condition and scheduling appointments if you keep your own records. Keep and file hard copies of all appointment records, tests ordered, test results, drug information, and office and doctor contact details, and keep CDs of scans.

▶ *Initiate Calls to Medical Records and to Your Doctor's Office*
If you call the medical records office at the hospital that did your tests, you can get your test results faster than waiting for the doctor's office to fill you in at your next appointment. If you want test-result interpretations before a scheduled appointment, call the doctor's office and request a phone call from your doctor. Most doctors—but not all, as I learned—will call you back.

▶ *Keep a Calendar of Symptoms*
Cancer treatment causes a host of reactions. You think you'll remember experiencing pain or other strange happenings, but at some point, things blur and it's very difficult to specifically track what you are experiencing and when. Keep a calendar, hard-copy or electronic, and capture how you are feeling and the associated symptoms. It will help guide discussions with your medical team, give you confidence in what you are saying, and help you and your doctors spot patterns that can perhaps be treated better or differently.

In summary, here are five things you can do to take action on knowing your medical history:

1. Know that HIPAA protects your rights for you to have your own medical records.
2. Start your own medical-history file folder.
3. Ask for and obtain hard copies of each medical report, scan, X-ray, or other test result and keep them in your file.
4. If needed, contact the medical-records department at your hospital yourself to obtain medical records.
5. Keep your own calendar of pain and how you feel on a day-by-day basis, noting any specific changes or symptoms.

CHAPTER 6:

Make Your List of Questions

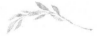

My mission is to enlighten people to a whole other way of thinking and approaching our health, which isn't necessarily driven by big business profit or a brainwashing that these doctors have had since medical school of how you're supposed to act with no radical thinking of asking other questions or considering that there's another way to solve a problem.

—FRAN DRESCHER, CANCER SURVIVOR AND ACTOR

A recent article in *Time* magazine notes that "asking questions is one of the best ways to ensure you and your doctor are on the same page. And if your doctor doesn't seem interested in answering, or you get a negative response, you need to find a new doctor."[1] My personal experiences exemplify this statement, and, yes, it may result in having to make drastic changes like finding a new doctor, but I assure you, it's for the better.

Have you asked questions of your doctor? If your answer is yes, that's good news. You are making the most out of your doctor visits. You're also in the minority.

For many people, the answer is "never," or at least "not nearly enough." Asking questions in any situation can be perceived in several ways—as curiosity, as engagement, and as doubt. But in a healthcare situation, you'd think that people would want to know more about their condition and ask many questions. Despite the many available tools and resources that provide lists of questions, and perhaps despite gut feelings that say "ask," questions are rarely verbalized.

Even in emergency medical situations, questions aren't asked. In a study published in the *Annals of Emergency Medicine*, emergency medicine physicians at Northwestern University's Feinberg School of Medicine looked at patients' understanding in four areas: diagnosis, treatment in the ER, instructions for at-home care, and hospital-discharge instructions. This study concluded that "78 percent of the 140 patients questioned did not understand instructions for their care after leaving the emergency room."[2] Another study found that 75 percent of doctors believed that they communicated satisfactorily with their patients, but only 21 percent of the people treated by those doctors said that their talks went well. In fact, according to the Agency for Healthcare Research and Quality, if a doctor asks a patient, "Do you have any questions?" the answer is almost always no.

Good communication, including asking questions, can impact a patient's understanding of the situation as well as real health outcomes. If questions can foster a better level of understanding and affect your health, why are patients so reticent to ask questions about their own health and walk away not understanding what needs to be done? Like with "speaking up," there are a variety of reasons.

Obstacles to Asking Questions

According to an article published by the US National Library of Medicine at the National Institutes for Health, patient literacy plays a role. "Although patient participation in the medical encounter confers significant benefits, many patients are reluctant to ask questions of their physicians. Patients' literacy level, [meaning their ability to read], may affect their level of participation and question-asking behaviors."[3] In the case of this particular study, the results concluded that adults with lower literacy levels ask statistically fewer questions than patients with high literacy levels.

Even when it comes to people with higher literacy levels, doctors, for the most part, have more medical knowledge and experience than their patients. Complex medical terms can stump even those who are highly literate. In reaction to medical-speak, many patients simply don't know what to ask or are embarrassed by the thought of sounding stupid. Or, conversely, patients may not want to risk aggravating their doctor, which may lead to less than the best care, so they trade their questions for silence. None of these behaviors help.

My research revealed a host of other reasons as well. Many people were raised with the idea that a doctor knows best and if there is something the doctor wants the patient to know, he or she will proactively say it. Questioning can also be viewed as doubting a doctor's judgment or ability.

In many doctor's appointments, doctors do most of the talking, and patients don't want to interrupt and then may forget a question that has popped up. With the time that doctors can spend with each patient being dictated by insurance, patients also can feel rushed and like there is not enough time for their questions or input when the doctor talking is more time sensitive.

Studies also show that often doctors don't ask, or don't ask in an effective way, if patients have questions. When asked, "Do you have any questions?" most patients will answer, "No." But studies show that when doctors ask questions differently—like "What questions do you have for me?" or "What can I do to help you better understand?"—patients start to think that they should have questions and feel more open to asking.

In a situation like cancer, just having to think or talk about your condition can cause immense anxiety. Fear of what a doctor may say plays a very real role in asking, or not asking, questions. That "ignorance is bliss" mentality is an easier route than asking the tough questions. But whether you ask or not, you will still have to face and deal with it. I chose to know what I was getting into, which helped me prepare and feel more in control. That serious feeling of lack of control is a major driver of anxiety and fear. Until you've been told that you, or a loved one, has cancer, you can't know the sense of fear that I mean.

Stacy

....

Looking back on this entire journey brings very conflicted feelings. Now that we are "done," I certainly do not have the same negative and petrifying feelings that I had initially . . . but I can still remember them. When you are told your child has cancer, what in my mind equated to a death sentence, you are immediately overcome with emotion. You can feel the dread washing through your body and landing in your gut as a nagging dull ache you just can't shake. And the fear. I have been scared before, like most people. Watching a horror movie, almost having an accident of some type, or maybe even seeing your young child take a harder-than-normal tumble. But this fear was different. This is the real deal. I have never felt so scared in my entire life. You can never really understand what it's like unless you're in the same position. Certainly, throughout my adult life, friends, colleagues, and acquaintances have all had trials and tribulations of some type where I tried to empathize with them. Back then I thought I was doing a good job. Little did I know I had no idea. How could I? Many people throughout this journey, especially in the

*beginning, would say things like, "I can imagine how this
feels." No, they really can't. This is a feeling you cannot understand unless it is real and happening to you. But I don't hold
it against them! How could they know? And I was just like
them, too, BC (before cancer).*

The fear is real with cancer.

That fear can serve as a disincentive to asking questions and
getting the information you need to feel in control and move forward.
According to the Harvard Medical School, it's tough to ask questions,
but "it can be even harder to disagree with healthcare providers, or
make known your worries and preferences for care." It's such a problem
that several organizations have created campaigns specifically aimed
at helping people talk more openly with their doctors."[4]

Help in Preparing Questions

If asking questions is important to your health outcomes, then what
questions should be asked? There are many online resources that provide guidance.

After the initial shock of a diagnosis, WebMD recommends taking
a course of action that includes taking control, finding a partner to consistently help you, getting organized, getting informed via seeking out
credible sources of information, and considering a second opinion.[5]

For example, the Agency for Healthcare Research and Quality
offers its "10 Questions You Should Know" materials.[6] The campaign
is based on the idea that doctors "know a lot about a lot of things, but
they don't always know everything about you or what is best for you."
With a list of ten general questions you should ask, the website also
provides questions to ask before, during, and after appointments. I
like that it's also customizable, with an interactive page that lets you
build your own list of questions. This kind of basic approach can help

a patient get grounded and think about how diagnosis and treatment will impact his or her life. Here are some sample questions:

1. What is the test for?
2. How many times have you done this procedure?
3. When will I get the results?
4. Why do I need this treatment?
5. Are there any alternatives?

I prepared for each doctor's appointment by doing my research—online and with knowledgeable contacts—and by writing down my questions in my healthcare notebook. By capturing the questions and answers in writing, I could refer to questions asked at past appointments and refresh my memory on answers or follow-up items.

Of course, I had questions about my condition, the course of treatment, side effects, and, if a test was run, test results. I also then always asked for a copy to be made of the test results for my personal medical-history file. Typically, I'd let the doctor brief me first. I'd ask questions as they naturally came up in the conversation, and then I checked my question list at the end to ensure I'd asked everything. If a question popped up and I did not want to interrupt the flow, I kept my notebook on my lap during the appointment and jotted down questions to ask afterward. This approach, my friends, takes preparation and work and is worth every bit of it.

You'll want to know the specifics about your condition, treatment, and follow-up, of course. Other questions will depend on what's important to you as a person. Here's where it's important to think about yourself, what you need, and what your instincts are telling you. Everyone is going to be a bit different. That's OK. You need to find the best fit for *you*, not for someone else.

Try to be clear about your individual needs, wants, and preferences. Some people may be comfortable with a big-name doctor because he or she has a great reputation for a certain specialty, and they may be willing to forgo a personal touch and convenient location. Someone else may need local care. Yet another may think it's important to have a personal referral from a friend or family member. There is no right or wrong; there's just what's right for you. Whatever is right for you, ask related questions to help you gauge what you need.

Here is a list of the questions I routinely asked, in addition to the specifics regarding any treatment and tests. I would go on to ask this same set of questions while getting a second opinion. (For more about that, see the next chapter, "Get a Second Opinion.")

1. Medically, what is my condition?
2. What steps do I need to take next?
3. What are the implications, and what big changes should I expect, i.e. time off work, major side effects, ability to care for family, etc.?
4. What are my options? (Note: there are always options, though they may not be offered unless you ask.)
5. What's a normal lifestyle at this point? Eating? Exercise? Travel? (My business requires me to travel, so ability to travel by car, plane, and train are essential for me.)
6. How can I promote recovery, naturally? (Note: natural recovery options are rarely offered, and you may need to seek answers through integrative medicine or on your own.)
7. What medications are you prescribing? What is the regimen, and what are the side effects?
8. What's the next course of treatment?
9. Who oversees my care? What are the names of the people on my medical team?
10. What are the recommended next steps?
11. How long will insurance approval take?

With surgery, I'd add:

1. How often do you perform this type of surgery?
2. How long will I be in the hospital? (Note: I took the answer to be a challenge and aimed to be out sooner.)
3. How can I avoid opioids?
4. Is there a fast track for recovery (Note: there usually is, but doctors may not talk about it unless you ask.)
5. Who is on call while I'm in the hospital? (Note: you want the doctor who performed the surgery to be available.)
6. When is the best time for this surgery to be scheduled? Will you or my other doctors be available or on call postoperatively? If the surgery is right before a holiday, will many members of your staff be off work? (Note: I avoided surgery before holidays when doctors were on vacation.)

The Silver-Bullet Question

In addition to these questions, the question I mentioned previously (about the doctor's cell phone number) was a "make or break" question that I asked of all the doctors I saw. "Can I have your cell phone number?" It was an unexpected question for them, but I've come to use it as a standard for whether a doctor is right for me. The question was important to me, not because I planned to call the doctor on his or her cell phone on a regular basis, but because it was a sign, to me, of the doctor's willingness to be available should I need him or her. The responses varied widely and told me everything *I* needed to know.

I'd save the question for last, after I was able to gather all the true medical details and get to know the doctor a bit. When I needed the colectomy surgery, the GI doctor who performed my colonoscopy referred me to a local experienced surgeon with a great reputation. I met with him and his nurses for a presurgical interview.

My questions revealed that he performed colectomy surgeries several times a month. Due to vacation schedules, the recommendation was that my surgery occur on the Friday before Memorial Day. In asking who would be on call, I found out that neither the surgeon nor the assisting surgeon would be in town over the holiday when I'd be recovering in the hospital.

The schedule was already giving me pause. Then I asked about him giving me his cell phone number. His answer, as I mentioned before, was, "I don't give out my number." I said, "If I really feel I need it, would you provide it?" The answer was, "If you really need it." *Hmm. I'm about to go through my first major surgery, related to cancer, and the surgeon will be out of town for my recovery and prefers to be unreachable?* That situation did not work for me, though I didn't think I had much of a choice, so I booked the surgery date.

A lesson to remember: you always have a choice.

Asking questions is a critically important tool in your medical-advocacy toolbox. Don't let intimidation, fear, lack of knowledge, or medical illiteracy deter you. Prepare and ask!

Anna

....

I was always fond of the phrase "How will you know unless you ask?" What I didn't know was how crucial that sentiment would become when faced with months of grueling treatments for cancer. Many times, what kept me going was the prospect of a family trip to Europe after the treatments were over. The problem was that the treatments had already robbed me of all of my energy. I had developed anemia, which exacerbated the fatigue, and I was afraid of not having enough time to recover to be able to enjoy the trip. I decided to help myself by asking my oncologist if we could decrease the time between my chemo sessions so as to finish the treatments earlier, thus giving me more time to recuperate. I presented my doctor with the plan, and much to my delight he agreed to the new schedule. I finished my treatments a week earlier than initially planned, giving me more valuable time to regain my strength. If he had said no, I would have accepted my fate, but not being afraid to ask proved not only to be beneficial but also uplifting. You should never be afraid to ask.

Taking Action on Making Your List of Questions

▶ *Do Your Homework in Advance of a Doctor's Appointment*
Knowledge is power! Being informed, educated, and prepared will help improve your sense of control and ability to communicate with your medical team. As you prepare, by using online tools and resources and talking with knowledgeable contacts, keep your notebook handy to jot down thoughts and questions.

▶ *Keep a Running List of Questions*
Cancer had a way of hogging up its unfair share of my mind. I found myself at times mentally consumed, almost constantly thinking about my condition. When I had a question, I wrote it down in my notebook. It relieved my mind, and it was in writing for my next appointment or call.

▶ *Use Available Resources to Get You Started*
If you don't even know where to start, or can't wrap your head around asking questions, use online resources to get you started. You can take a look at the resources named in this chapter or simply google "What questions should I ask my doctor?" and a host of resources will pop up for your review. It's really that easy to find volumes of helpful

information. Or add a bit more specificity to it and Google, "What questions should I ask at my first oncology appointment?"

▶ *Consider What's Important to You*
Prewritten questions from online resources can provide a great jump start for the medical approach, but give some careful consideration to what's important and meaningful to you. A doctor's personal touch? His or her being best in class? Convenience? Once you know what's important to you, be sure to include some questions that help you get at those answers.

▶ *Ask for the Cell Phone Number*
(or write your own make-or-break question):
After sorting through medical capabilities, my make-or-break question was "Can I have your cell phone number?" This question worked for me as a final and determining filter, even though I ultimately never called my doctors on their cell phones. Pick your make-or-break question, and don't be afraid to ask it!

In summary, here are five things you can do to take action on making your list of questions:

1. Do your homework in advance of your doctor's appointment.
2. Keep a running list of questions in your medical file folder.
3. Use available resources to get your list of questions started.
4. Consider what's most important to *you*.
5. Ask for the doctor's cell phone number.

CHAPTER 7:

Get a Second Opinion

I asked, "Will it kill me?" His frighteningly cavalier response of "Well, it's cancer" sent a chill down my spine and made me realize that I needed to advocate for myself. My first step was to get a new doctor! You have to trust your gut and know that not all doctors are created equal.
—KERRY KENNA, CANCER SURVIVOR
AND PATIENT ADVOCATE

How many dresses or pairs of shoes do we try on until we find the "right" one for the occasion? How many cars do we test drive before we pick the model we'll buy? How many reviews or recommendations do we read before we place an order for a simple who knows what on Amazon?

If you have a lawyer, accountant, public relations firm, plumber, financial advisor, or any other service provider and you aren't completely satisfied with their work or sure about them, you seek another. Options and getting second opinions are a regular part of our daily lives in almost any situation. So why is it in healthcare that getting a second opinion feels so tough and uncomfortable?

According to Harvard Health Publishing, 70 percent of Americans don't feel compelled to get a second opinion or do additional research.[1] Prior to going through something as serious as cancer treatment, this figure probably would not have shocked me. But, after firsthand experience in seeing how important the right medical provider for each patient can be, it's astounding.

Beyond getting a second opinion to find the best medical fit for you, a recent study by Mayo Clinic researchers suggests that patients who get second opinions often receive different diagnoses. Of the 286 cases in this study, 21 percent resulted in a different diagnosis and, in 66 percent of the cases, the diagnosis was better defined or refined.[2]

Stacy

I advise all cancer patients to seek a second opinion at an NCI-Designated Cancer Center (https://www.cancer.gov/research/infrastructure/cancer-centers). I realize that social determinants of health, inequities, and disparities can make this challenging. I am hopeful that with the accelerated adoption of telemedicine by COVID-19, we can make this more readily possible. Generally, cancer treatment protocols are methodical, but the second opinion may be to find a clinical trial, try an innovative new drug combo or technology, and/or deem a patient a surgical candidate when thought otherwise. The oncology/surgical team usually requires imaging, radiology reports, pathology reports, doctor-visit notes, hospitalizations, patient history, family history, blood work, tumor markers (CEA, CA-125, etc.), and prior treatments. Gathering this information and transmitting it can be cumbersome, hence the optimism around electronic means. Also, patients need to first check with their insurance carriers to confirm reimbursement policies around second opinions. Do not feel uncomfortable or intimidated to pursue a second opinion. It is merely more eyes looking at your case to provide more information and expertise. My biggest success story of a second opinion was a patient named Kevin with neuroendocrine cancer. Kevin was relentless in pushing to three different institutions until he felt confident he was receiving the best, most up-to-date care. He is outlasting his less-than-ten-percent odds and is currently living a full, survivor, thriver life.

Obstacles to Getting Second Opinions

Still, patients are generally reluctant to get or ask their physicians for a second opinion. Beyond reluctance, getting a second opinion is simply not the norm, based on national data, and based on the many conversations I have had on the topic with patients of all types. Most people accept the first physician that is assigned or recommended to them, and most people accept the treatment plan that the physician recommends.

My question is, why? Why are most patients so seemingly accepting and not requesting a second opinion with cancer care that will absolutely be a life-changing experience, most of which is highly unpleasant? Research—mine and that of many others—shows that there are several main reasons for not seeking a second opinion.

First, many people don't want to challenge the doctor's judgment or make the doctor think that he or she is not trusted. Patients think it could signal a lack of confidence in the physician's credibility.

Next, many patients don't want to seem rude or insulting and potentially damage their relationship with the doctor. Nor do patients also want to be perceived as difficult. Not having your doctor "like" you could impact the type of care you receive.

Because medical offices are so busy, asking for a second opinion is perceived to create more work for an already-overburdened staff. And, truthfully, it creates more work and time commitment from the patient, who is already spending an inordinate amount of time in medical facilities.

In my case, the time involved with getting a second opinion gave me pause. Back to my friend who had the double-mastectomy: she actively sought a second opinion, even though it took some additional time to do. But guess what? The opinions varied greatly on the recommended course of action. In the end, it was her decision on how to proceed, but the second opinion gave her much more information with which to make her decision.

Given the high expense of medical appointments, cost also crosses the minds of patients when thinking about a second opinion. In doing research for this book, I learned that most health plans seem to cover the cost of a second opinion in cases that are serious and life-threatening, but be sure to check with your insurance provider if cost is a concern.

Some patients believe that doctors won't disagree with each other, so getting a second opinion would result in the same diagnosis or approach. As cited earlier, second opinions often conflict with first opinions and may result in a more refined approach. In my case, the course of treatment was very similar, but my comfort level with the medical teams was very different, which I would not have known with only one opinion.

Finally, and sadly, others think that perhaps there is no hope, no matter who is treating them and what the treatment is, so they accept the first opinion because they think nothing else will really help.

It's interesting to note that most of these reasons, cost excluded, are not patient-centered. The patient is putting the doctor—their feelings, ego, and judgment—at the center of the decision-making. If patients don't put themselves at the center of their own care, then how can we expect our healthcare system to be truly patient-centered?

At the end of the day, I think it comes down to this: after working through the objections and considering all the good reasons to seek a second opinion, it still just feels uncomfortable. Cancer patients are already uncomfortable in so many ways that adding to the discomfort is not something they want to do. But it's worth the time and discomfort to push for a second opinion.

In my experience, the first surgeon recommended to me had great experience and credentials, but something didn't feel right, as I noted earlier. Getting a second opinion for surgery was time-consuming, at a time when time was of the essence, and felt a little like I was betraying the first surgeon. In fact, the diagnosis and treatment were almost identical. But through his experience and personality, the second surgeon gave me so much more confidence that I can't help but think it helped me in the procedure and recovery.

Getting a Referral or Recommendation

The way I handled getting this second opinion was completely divorced from the first surgeon and hospital. I sought recommendations from family and friends and independently pursued an appointment and opinion from a second provider at a completely different hospital. Once my surgery was scheduled with the second doctor, I called the office of the first surgeon, thanked them for talking with me, told them I found a surgeon who performed the procedure much more often and with whom I felt comfortable.

With my postoperative chemo treatment, an oncologist was recommended by my surgeon, whom I trusted. The oncologist was smart, capable, and experienced, and I liked him. He gave me the option of receiving chemo at the facility where he worked or at a satellite facility much closer to my home. Given how much I'd need to travel, I selected the satellite one closest to me.

The oncologist at the satellite facility who would oversee my treatment just didn't feel right to me from the start. Since my course of treatment had been designed by the first oncologist whom I trusted, I thought things would be OK. As it turned out, after about a month, my body violently rejected the treatment and things went downhill fast. Though I had reported my decline and had been calling the satellite oncologist's office, not much was being done to help.

After speaking up for myself, getting the help of local chemo-center nurses, and going back to consult with the original, non-satellite, oncologist, the treatment got back on course. I am quite certain that if I had not forced action to receive a second opinion on a chemo-treatment correction, I would have physically and mentally collapsed.

Ovie

Research the cancer centers, travel if you have to, and get a second opinion. I was diagnosed with a genetic breast cancer, BRCA1, triple negative, at thirty-nine. This was a concern as I had lost my mother, sister, and two aunts to cancer. I refused to be treated as a routine cancer patient, and I found a doctor at Sloan Kettering to review my case. This doctor's specialty was dealing with aggressive cancer. I believe this was crucial in my treatment plan and for my survival.

While it may cause discomfort to get a second opinion, the stats show that it's worth it. It's your health. You owe it to yourself. You are worth a second opinion.

Taking Action on Getting a Second Opinion

▶ *Be Upfront*

Be honest, forthcoming, and kind from the beginning. Let the doctor know that cancer, or any life-threatening condition, is scary and that you take comfort in hearing a variety of opinions, so you're talking with them as well as with at least one other. The conversation does not have to have a mean or demeaning tone. Perhaps that doctor has a recommendation for someone else you could talk to. I preferred going to a different hospital system so I could get a truly different opinion. If a doctor balks at your approach, they are not the right doctor for you. WebMD suggests that you *should* tell your doctor that you are seeking a second opinion for a very practical reason because it will be easier to share records and information between practices if all doctors are in the know. However, if you employ my approach of being the keeper of your medical records, you are free to pursue care and opinions with your records readily available. If you are completely uncomfortable being open, seek a second opinion on your own without discussing it with the first doctor. Just be sure you have all your necessary records. It would be polite to round back with the doctor with whom you won't be moving forward with and let him or her know you'll be treated elsewhere. If you prefer to have specific questions to guide your conversation, the American Cancer Society, as well as other online resources, provide guidelines in seeking a second opinion. They include questions like:

- "I'm thinking of getting a second opinion. Can you recommend someone?"
- "Before we start treatment, I'd like to get a second opinion. Will you help me with that?"

- "If you had my type of cancer, is there another doctor you would see for a second opinion?"

▶ *Ask Friends and Family*

If you are at a loss for where to find a second opinion, my first suggestion is to ask for recommendations from friends and family. There's nothing like a firsthand experience or testimony.

▶ *Use Hospital Resources*

The websites for hospitals also provide information on doctors and specialists of all types. You can identify doctors via those online tools and then look at online reviews for just about any doctor.

▶ *Telemedicine*

With the growth of telemedicine, especially since COVID-19, there are now online services available that provide second opinions. And, since COVID-19 accelerated the use of telemedicine in general, many, though not all, doctors are amenable to telehealth visits that can be done via phone or video call. I've not used any of these services, but as the telemedicine industry grows, it will no doubt be faster and easier to obtain a second opinion, though trust may come into play with online offerings.

▶ *It's Your Right*

Second opinions help you learn more about your condition and diagnosis. Just like in life, doctors range from conservative to aggressive. Treatment and technology also vary from hospital to hospital. What's good for someone else may not be good for you. It's your right, as a patient with a serious illness, to get a second opinion. Cut yourself a break and use your rights. It's OK to find what's best for you.

In summary, here are six things you can do to take action and get a second opinion:

1. Be upfront and ask your doctor for a recommendation for a second opinion.
2. Seek recommendations from family and friends.
3. Use hospital websites and online reviews to review physician options and ratings.
4. Use online resources to help guide the conversation with your doctor.
5. Consider telemedicine options for interviewing second opinions.
6. Remember, a second opinion is your right.

CHAPTER 8:

Prepare for Treatment

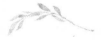

Like with every form of cancer, early detection is what it's all about. I urge everyone to learn about this condition. It can be prevented with testing and can be beaten if caught early.
—ROD STEWART, CANCER SURVIVOR
AND ONE OF MY FAVORITE SINGERS

Prior to cancer, my only real experience with something surgical was delivering two babies, which I approached like an athlete in training. My thought process was that if I was in the best shape possible, mentally and physically, then I'd give myself the best chance to have easier deliveries. Eating right, daily exercise, massage, relaxation, and happy thoughts served as my daily routine. There were a few scares and detours along the way, but my pregnancies were relatively easy, and my body snapped back post-pregnancy (though there are some things that will remain unsaid and are permanently different!).

When I got the news and came to the realization that I needed to have a colectomy (a surgery that would remove almost a foot of my large colon), that same "training" instinct kicked in. Maybe it's because my dad was a drill instructor in the Marine Corps, but surgical preparation became my mission.

There was about a month between my colonoscopy/diagnosis and the surgery, and I used that time to eat as nutritiously as possible and to exercise so that my body would be in the best shape possible. A strong mind supports a strong body, so mental preparedness was also key. Having no real idea of what I was in for, I did my best to prepare.

In preparing for surgery, and later when living through treatment, there were two key areas, in particular, where I made serious assumptions that turned out to be untrue and are worth calling out for readers.

One: Approaching a patient's healing and recovery is holistic, in my opinion. As mentioned previously, food, exercise, lifestyle, medical treatment, and medicine all work together. This approach, however, is not commonly used in our healthcare system.

The medical team primarily focuses on medicine, as in pharmaceutical drugs as the first-line and sometimes only solution, unless you ask, probe, and integrate other solutions for lifestyle changes, supplementation, exercise, and holistic solutions on your own. Perhaps it's a blinding glimpse of the obvious, but healthcare is not about healthcare; it's about treating lack of health with drugs.

Two: When you watch medical advertising and marketing, it looks convincing, even to someone, like me, who is a marketer. Hospitals tout new research, science, and high-tech labs and show how personalized medicine works to cure celebrities like local football heroes. My experience showed me quite another side, where, sadly, the realities of science have not caught up with medical marketing.

Cancer treatment, in many cases, is a numbers game. It is not personalized like the marketing would lead you to believe. It is based on clinical trials with people who may not be anything like you and with drugs that were approved years ago.

The initial chemo regimen that was proposed for me was 5-FU, which was initially studied in the 1950s and in clinical trials in the 1980s! Seriously, that's nearly forty years ago. Believe it or not, that regimen is what one of my oncologists still predominantly recommends. Xeloda, the oral chemotherapy drug I was on, was approved by the FDA in 2001. Oxaliplatin, the chemo infusion drug I received, was approved by the FDA in 2004, with clinical trials happening years before then. Many other cancer drugs were approved prior to 2000. Drug approval is a long and careful process, but come on, people, these treatments are older than most of the technology we use on a daily basis! One would think there are more progressive treatments, but these dated ones are still the accepted standards.

While clinical trials are certainly a gold standard for safety and efficacy, these commonly used drugs are dated, which stands in stark contrast to the medical marketing that leads you to believe you will receive the latest and greatest in science and personalized medicine.

As you prepare for surgery, keep in mind that your holistic health will be *your* responsibility. Most surgeons and cancer doctors and medical teams have not studied nutrition or integrative therapies and are not in a position, oddly enough, to help you. Seek out resources in advance so you can incorporate lifestyle, nutrition, exercise, and supplementation changes with as much time as possible for them to have a positive impact—things like meditation to keep a clear mind, walking to build stamina, and supplements that help deter inflammation.

When surgery and postsurgical treatment plans are discussed, be sure to research them and understand if they really are the best solution for you and your circumstances, not just the most common and accepted, and perhaps dated, courses of treatment. For example, when discussing surgery with the first surgeon, he suggested that he and a colleague do the procedure together and use a robot, an emerging technology, to assist. I liked the idea of using the most up-to-date technology, but then I came to find out through research that my body shape (relatively small) and location of the part of the colon that needed to be removed would have prevented the mobility of the robot.

I also opted, in advance, for a nonopioid postsurgical recovery plan, with pain management using only Tylenol. While in the hospital, I walked the halls as much as possible to jump-start my physical recovery while still under medical supervision.

In addition to preparing for treatment with medical input, connecting with someone who has had a similar diagnosis can be very helpful. Understanding the experience of another person, from a patient perspective, not from a medical perspective, can provide comfort as well as information.

Andrea

When I was first diagnosed, I was contacted by an old friend who I had been in touch with off and on but who I had not seen for a while. She had heard I had been diagnosed, and she wanted to reach out to support me as she herself had just completed treatment for breast cancer. As it turned out, we had the same type of cancer and almost identical treatment plans. Because she had recently been through it, she was able to provide me some amazing insights on what to expect, what to ask my doctor, and how to best navigate the entire process. She told me about how to prepare for chemo and what to have on hand at home. She encouraged me to ask my doctor about potential side effects. Every step along the way, she was able to provide information that helped me navigate my journey. This isn't for everyone, but my advice is to seek out those with a similar diagnosis. Their firsthand experience, while maybe different from yours, can help you to understand your options and help you to form questions that you can ask your doctor.

Of course this is all about information, not advice. Many organizations, like the American Cancer Society, are able to connect patients. ACS's program called Reach To Recovery pairs newly diagnosed breast cancer patients with survivors who have been trained to share information and provide resources. The patients are paired based on similar treatment/ diagnosis. For example, someone who is HER2 positive and will receive chemo and radiation. Many women have various questions before radiation, such as "Will I be able to wear a bra during treatment?" This is a question that comes up from women who continue to work during treatment. I am a trained R To R volunteer.

Food as Medicine

Preparing for surgery can be approached from both physical and mental perspectives, and both are important. If you look online, you can find dozens of "checklists" of how to prepare for surgery. Things like "wear comfortable clothes" and "have someone to drive you home" are frequently mentioned. My focus is not on the nuts and bolts of what clothes to pack, but rather what you can do to help you optimize your physical and mental condition so that you can get your life back to normal as soon as possible.

I am a big believer that you are what you eat, and that food plays a central role in healing, so nutrition became a focus for me. My research led me to focus on an anti-inflammatory diet. My typical daily diet consisted of the following:

Breakfast: granola, fresh fruit, and coffee
Supplements: women's multivitamin pack and turmeric
Midmorning snack: fruit and peanut butter, peanut butter bar, or almonds

Lunch: yogurt or smoothie with yogurt, fruit, greens, honey, turmeric, and ginger

Dinner: salad, preferably with kale, beets, garbanzo beans, a piece of organic chicken or salmon, and homemade olive oil and vinegar dressing

Water: about ninety ounces a day. (Naturally flavored sparkling water and kombucha are pretty much the only other beverages I drank.)

Things that I love that I minimized: breads, pastas, chocolate, pizza

Things that I occasionally enjoy that I pretty much gave up: red meat of all kinds, any food or product with added sugars, fruit juices

Things that I never included in my diet: fast food of any kind, soda, alcohol, highly processed foods

I also continued this diet post-surgery, as much as possible. Immediately after surgery, I was on a liquid and then soft, low-roughage diet, so I included chicken-broth-based homemade soups.

Immediate post-surgery food, while still in the hospital, was a concern to me. How many times have you visited someone in the hospital only to see them being fed Salisbury steak, Jell-O, and packaged lemonade? Those items were certainly not included in my postoperative diet.

What was brought to me post-surgery was even more shocking. Colon surgery dictates a liquid diet. My food tray consisted of a variety of sugar- and salt-laden liquids, including packaged iced tea, Jell-O, bouillon-cube broth, and other assorted liquid-sugar substances (I wish I'd had the presence of mind to snap a photo).

Hello? Cancer feeds on sugar, and my recovery meals basically consisted of liquid sugar. Fortunately, the thought of Salisbury steak and mashed potatoes scared me to the point that I had prepared my own, grandma's recipe, homemade chicken soup. We brought it with us when we came in for surgery, and the nice nurses kept it in a nearby refrigerator in my unit. That soup, and water, kept me going and served as my meals until I could eat more solid food.

Given my shock and dismay over the contents of the liquid diet, I did request to talk with someone from hospital nutrition, but no one showed up in my room to talk. I did note my nutritional concerns on the postoperative survey, though again, no feedback.

In the chemo center, many patients' treatments take hours. If you are there for the better part of the day, you get hungry. Snacks were offered in the chemo center that I went to. Those snacks, as you may have guessed at this point, were processed cookies and crackers full of sugar, high-fructose corn syrup, and sodium. Here we were, trying to cure ourselves of all types of cancers with expensive, time-consuming drugs, and what we were offered to put into our bodies was just what we shouldn't be.

Once I started chemo, two months after surgery, nothing tasted right. I developed "aversions" to some of my go-to foods like kale, coffee, and peanut butter. With these aversions, even the thought of these foods I'd once loved made me incredibly sick, and I had to avoid them. I wouldn't wish them on my worst enemy. Happily, most of them are back into my regular diet.

The healthcare system must reevaluate its approach to food as medicine, too, and educate and serve healing, nutritious food as part of treatment. But until they do, consider it your responsibility as a patient to research and tend to your personal nutritional needs.

Exercise

Exercise was also an important component of my presurgical training, as it is for maintaining an optimal quality of life in general. Being in shape prior to treatment makes it easier to bounce back after surgery or treatment. Always one to exercise regularly, I ramped up my usual time and effort spent exercising in order to get myself in optimum physical shape, for me. Here was my weekly exercise routine:

Monday: one-hour step aerobics class at gym, followed by weight lifting for upper body
Tuesday: one-hour hot yoga class
Wednesday: walk three miles or stair stepper
Thursday: one-hour step aerobics class followed by weightlifting for lower body
Friday: one-hour hot yoga class
Saturday: one-hour hot yoga class or walk three miles
Sunday: walk three miles

The combination of cardio, weight training, stretching, and mindful walking worked well for me. There was enough variety to keep my interest and to develop all-around physical fitness. This work-out routine was like the one I had been doing the year before I was diagnosed, but I ramped up the intensity and frequency so that I was doing something daily. Post-surgery and during chemo, my work-out routine was forced to change dramatically.

In talking with other women who have undergone cancer treatment, I learned that quite a few others took a similar approach, with physical training and a focus on nutrition, and found it helpful in both dealing with the cancer diagnosis as well as the treatment and recovery.

Stacy

I am currently in my fifth year of achieving no evidence of disease (NED) status in surviving stage IV colorectal cancer. I had a 14 percent chance of getting this far, so I feel extraordinarily fortunate. I'm often asked how I did it. I got ANTSY against cancer (Attitude, Nutrition, Treatment, Support, You)! First, I maintained a positive, can-do mindset. Second, I adopted a mainly plant-based diet based on "foods that fight cancer" recommended by the American Institute for Cancer Research (https://www.aicr.org/cancer-prevention/food-facts/?gclid =EAIaIQobChMIooX9tcaL6gIVAuDICh2SNQOX EAAYASAAEgLWX_D_BwE). I also eliminated sugar, fried foods, dairy, processed meat, and alcohol. Third, I assembled a collaborative, best-in-class medical team at an NCI-Designated Cancer Center whom I fully trusted and adored. I was supported by family and friends, and I researched both print and online resources in order to be my own best advocate and maintain my mental/emotional health. Finally, I maintained work and hobbies, which empowered me to feel "normal" and not let my existence become a "cancer patient."

It's Mental, as Well as Physical

Being a believer in the power of the mind, I did several things to try and keep my mind focused on positivity and gratitude, which is a true challenge when cancer enters your life. A lover of books, I read inspirational selections, including the Bible, *The Secret*, and books about harnessing your energy to heal.

Healing energy is a topic that sparked my interest. A recent *Forbes* article described healing energy this way: "Routinely touted as 'alternative medicine,' energy-based healing is, in fact, a centuries-old practice.... Although the various schools of thought differentiate slightly, it is generally accepted that energetic imbalances and disturbances to energy flow, even subtle, are the cause of maladies."[1]

Just a few months prior to my diagnosis, a friend told me about her positive experiences with a local energy healer and recommended trying it. I did, and interestingly, during the session, the energy healer asked me if I was having stomach issues, because he sensed some energy blockage in my lower abdomen. Just a few months later, I was diagnosed with colon cancer.

The treatments seemed to help me relax and restore balance, both physically and mentally, and I incorporated them into my health regime every few months—though I had to limit my energy healing treatments a bit during chemo because I could not sit through a one-hour car trip without having to use a bathroom. I believe in their power and try to incorporate energy healing practices into my daily life. You may be familiar with energy healing approaches like Reiki, craniosacral massage, universal energy healing, acupressure (which I have used for allergy-related sinus congestion), acupuncture, essential oil therapy, or others.

While I always thought of myself as grateful, I started a gratitude journal and wrote in it each night a list of things that I was grateful for that day, ranging from the love of family and having a working digestive system to sunshine and my cats. It's funny what you become grateful for when you have experienced the loss of it. The gratitude journal is a powerful tool and is something I practice even now.

Taking Action on Preparing for Treatment

▶ *Use a Combined Physical and Mental Approach*
Undergoing cancer treatment can be physically grueling, and if you start off in good physical shape, it will be easier to bounce back post-treatment. Use the time between diagnosis and treatment to get your body into as good of physical shape as you can muster. While physical conditioning helps, mental conditioning is just as important. Focus your mind on positive outcomes. The mind can have an amazing impact on your body and health.

▶ *Think about Food as Medicine*
I've heard it said that each bite of food you take is either promoting health or disease. When you are diagnosed with cancer, take this advice

to heart. Eat foods that promote health and enable your body to heal and recover. Skip foods and drinks that are high in sugar (a known promoter of cancer) or those that are known to be inflammatory. Food can be as healing as pharmaceuticals, and without side effects.

▶ *Consider Integrative Medicine in Addition to Traditional*

Natural and homeopathic solutions were helpful to me, and I preferred them to pharmaceuticals, which often have undesirable side effects. Seek out integrative medicine specialists in your area and get their recommendations. As telehealth has become more available, integrative medicine specialists may be more accessible to you for consults.

▶ *Don't Trust Hospital Food for Nutrition*

I can't answer why hospital food isn't nutritious and why it's not specific to healing. I do know that I was served a tray full of liquid sugar immediately after cancer surgery and that I didn't eat it. Being prepared by bringing my own homemade food with me to the hospital served me well.

▶ *Gratitude Is an Important Part of Treatment Prep*

While it's never easy to be grateful in the face of adversity, making mindful choices to be grateful for the many things I did have helped me navigate my cancer journey. Even now, I try to start each day with a gratitude meditation and a strong focus on the good that is currently in my life.

In summary, here are five things you can do to take action on preparing for treatment:

1. Help your body and mind get into the best physical and mental condition possible.

2. Use food as medicine.
3. Seek nutrition and integrative medical counsel and support.
4. Bring your own food to the hospital.
5. Be grateful.

CHAPTER 9:

Talk with Family and Friends (or Don't)

I've had two cancer bouts in my years on the court, and the first one, Justice O'Connor told me, "Now, you do the chemotherapy on Friday because you'll get over it during the weekend and you can be back in court on Monday."
—RUTH BADER GINSBURG, CANCER SURVIVOR
AND SUPREME COURT JUSTICE

In tough situations, family and friends can be incredibly supportive, kind, helpful, and motivational. My husband, kids, mom, and sister and a handful of dear friends were my close circle of trusted confidantes and strength. They almost always knew the right touch for me and were sensitive to me not wanting to share too much and too broadly.

In tough situations, family and friends can also say and do the most thoughtless, senseless, and hurtful things. It's amazing how sometimes those closest to you can be the least in touch with what would be most helpful or seem to not care at all. To be fair, no one, not even someone who has gone through cancer treatment, can really know what another cancer patient is going through. The disease, its treatment, and how your mind and body react are all very personalized.

Quite a few fellow cancer patients I have talked with echoed that friends and family can say the dumbest things. It's tough to know what to say, I guess, but it's much tougher being on the receiving end. During a recent webinar for cancer survivors, one of the topics that drew the most ire from survivors was "things that people say that really bother you." Comments like "My sister-in-law had cancer; I know just how you feel" (no, you don't), "Oh, that's not good," or "Will you lose all of your hair?" are just the tip of the stupidity iceberg.

Saying dumb things to people with cancer seems to be commonplace. According to an article published by CURE (Cancer Updates, Research, and Education), an organization that polled cancer patients, it's shockingly common. The CURE article featured commentary by Dan Gottlieb, PhD, a psychologist who hosts a long-running show on WHYY radio in Philadelphia. He did a recent segment in which he helped explain why people say such ridiculous things to those with cancer.

Some of the comments are thoughtless ("everything happens for a reason") and some are outright offensive ("I don't know how you can go to the grocery store with no hair"). While almost inconceivable that these types of things are said, they are, commonly. Dr. Gottlieb explains that our brains make us anxious with unfamiliar situations and that we instinctively try to assess if we are at risk. Those stupid things are said, on an unconscious level, to create distance from the person with cancer and to help the person that says them manage his or her own anxiety.

Dr. Gottlieb's advice? If you want to say something, just ask if you can help and how. And sometimes you don't have to say anything. "If you care, just care," he adds. "Often, you don't need words."[1]

Even as a cancer patient myself, I can't know what someone else is experiencing, and I never make assumptions. Just let someone know you care and are there for them.

If you encounter comments that strike you as dumb, careless, or just plain infuriating, you can give someone the benefit of the doubt and let it roll off, though this is not easy. You may need to avoid someone who repeatedly says the wrong things. Do what works for you so that you can focus on healing and recovery.

Silence, for me, was equally as disconcerting as a dumb comment. If someone was close enough to me to know about my condition but completely ignored it and never even asked how I was feeling, it felt devoid of caring altogether.

Sadly, sharing or talking about it can be awkward for cancer patients and for those around them, which is why some people choose to just keep the diagnosis to themselves. How and when people decide to share information about a serious illness or life-threatening condition is deeply personal.

Marie
....

My doctor recommended I have a hysterectomy after some testing showed I had precancerous cells in my uterus, which later turned to stage I uterine cancer. Of course, I turned to my two best girlfriends for advice and consolation, both of whom made me feel tremendous anxiety. One was flippant, because she'd had a hysterectomy, and said it was no big deal and to "go for it." Later, she projected her experience onto mine and, in trying to be there for me, ultimately tried to control my experience. The other was into alternative medicine and made me feel bad about considering traditional treatment; she made me highly anxious in every conversation. I know they were trying to help, but I found the most solace in advice from strangers and acquaintances, all of whom had friends or women in their families who had experienced similar issues. Opening up to people at some personal distance from me turned out to be the greatest gift.

The path I chose was one of keeping my cancer diagnosis and treatment very close to the vest. Everyone will be different, and it's worth thinking through how you or a loved one will handle communications if you are in a situation with a serious diagnosis.

Being a private person by nature, such a devastating diagnosis was not something I'd be inclined to disclose. Being in business, I didn't want any preconceived ideas about cancer to color my interactions with clients or other business connections. When I was working in the agency world, it was, and still is, a cutthroat business. I'd seen people become extremely vulnerable when associated with a serious condition—you could almost see the vultures circling. I witnessed that "illness" equated to being weak and learned not to be seen as vulnerable.

To be honest, telling people makes things more real, and, in some ways, by curtailing who knew, I could more easily go on with my normal life and not have to deal with questions and concern in most of my daily interactions. In many ways, keeping it to myself took the pressure off me.

In my mind, there were more pros than cons to keeping my diagnosis, surgery, and treatment details contained. There were, however, unexpected cons to my approach. In essence, there were times when I felt like I was living a lie, not being true to who I really was at that time. Trying to cover my weight loss, my inability to eat, and my pain and pretend like nothing was wrong was hard and inauthentic for me.

Just like any other information, once you tell someone, it's difficult to control the sharing and the narrative, and your condition can take on a life of its own. Many people, mostly younger, as research shows, prefer to be open and share details, especially with the help of social media.

Cancer "coming out" via social media is apparently a thing. While it may seem impersonal, it also has advantages. According to a story in the *Boston Globe*, Facebook and other social media do have some real advantages for communicating about health problems. Online communication doesn't take the emotional or physical energy of informing people in person or over the phone—and the news all goes out in one go.[2]

Beware, however, that social networks, like Facebook, harvest healthcare data with questionable security and, according to the Federal Trade Commission, "questionable ethics." The extent of Facebook's data collection is unclear, but we do know that Facebook collects preferences, and those preferences are used to serve up ads and content. The questions around health data privacy are important, though currently unanswered.

Only having to tell the story once is easier, less draining emotionally, and less time-consuming than repeating the same sad story over and over again. "On the plus side, you'll get immediate social support—from prayers to proffered meals to practical advice from others who've been there. It's efficient, immediate, and you don't have to have the same cancer conversation again and again," says a story on the topic in the Fred Hutch newsletter.

The same article notes that, "On the downside, you may also get crackpot theories about how you can cure cancer with baking soda or critiques about your treatment choices (this happens in the real world, too). Some people may post 'blamey' articles on your wall about the link between cancer and, say, processed meat (usually right beneath your Fourth of July barbecue pics). As with all things in life, Facebook can be a mixed bag."[3]

My Facebook cancer "coming out" was met with an avalanche of support, positivity, and caring. It was very helpful to me to be able to control what was said and when it was said—at a time of my choosing, when the cancer was already in treatment—and in a forum of friends, all at once.

Using social media to share a cancer diagnosis is not reserved for use by the young. My gosh, *Jeopardy* host Alex Trebek chose to share his diagnosis of Stage IV pancreatic cancer; he did so via Twitter, in a one-minute-and-thirteen-second videotaped message from the *Jeopardy* set.

Before you let the cancer cat out of the bag, or not, carefully consider what will work best for you. Once you go public, you can't take it back.

My dear friend Lisa Lurie, who penned the foreword for this book, took an interesting approach to her cancer communications. Not wanting to sap her precious energy needed for treatment and healing, she decided that her husband would serve as chief cancer communicator for her. Updates, phone calls, and other communication ran through him. When Lisa was recovering and feeling like she could resume communications on her own, she did.

With her amazing strength, she then, along with her cofounder, Ellen, started the organization Cancer Be Glammed. CBG provides women diagnosed with all forms of cancer with easy access to fashionable recovery products and lifestyle solutions. Talk about being a successful cancer communicator! Thank you, Lisa, for all you do.

Other friends used similar approaches that worked very well for them.

Andrea

I remember that days after my diagnosis, I started to receive calls from people wanting to talk and asking about my situation and how they could help. One day I had seventeen voicemails on my phone when I returned from a doctor appointment . . .

everyone saying, "Call me." It was overwhelming. I'd make one call back, and I was so emotionally drained that I couldn't respond to anyone else. The pressure to call someone back with updates was too much. My friend Amy volunteered to be my "voice" and created a blog where she and I could provide updates for those who wanted information or wanted to know how to help. Initially, she drafted the blog—I was too tired and sick to do so—based on my input, and then as I started to feel better, I updated the blog myself. It was a helpful way to keep everyone informed and for me to focus on getting better. My advice is to find someone who is willing to be your voice to share approved info and updates. And my advice to those who want to support patients, if you do call and need to leave a message, is to just say hello and let the person know you're thinking of them. Don't ask for a call back or how you can help—it can feel more like a burden than a nice interaction if the person is already feeling overwhelmed. A nice message or note goes a long way!

Telling the Kids

Adult family and friends are one thing, but if you have children, talking with them about cancer is quite another. Whoever thinks they will need to have such a discussion? Certainly not me. "Cancer" is such a scary word, associated with scary things, especially for kids. Few words strike more fear in anyone's heart.

I must say, of all my family and friends, our two kids, aged sixteen and thirteen at the time, handled the news better than anyone. To be honest, sharing the news with my kids is a blur. The weekend of my diagnosis was filled with tears and obvious upset. The kids, however, seemed unflappable.

Many guidelines say you should talk to kids about how their lives may change. The American Cancer Society suggests that the approach be adapted to the ages of the children but encourages sharing the type of cancer, the body part where the cancer is, how it will be treated, and how their lives will be affected.[4]

While I shared the first three items, throughout my journey, I tried my best not to let my condition impact them or change their lives. There were fewer homemade dinners and fewer school and sports events attended, but life went on. As I look back, except for coming to a few chemo treatments with me and visiting me in the hospital when I had surgery, their schedules and lives were unaffected in many ways.

What I remember well, however, is that they never seemed overly worried. Thank God for teenage centrism. Somehow, they never made comments or asked questions that seemed dumb or irritating. They were at the same time amazingly supportive and nonchalant. Their world continued, mostly as usual, and we worked hard to make it seem that way.

My at-the-time fourteen-year-old nephew was one of my biggest supporters during cancer treatment. He would come to many of my chemo infusions, along with my mom. No stranger to infusions himself, he would sit, chat, play video games, and just be there with me in a way that was more loving and supportive than most adults could. Just thinking about his loving support, without a single hint of complaining or grief, makes me cry.

In talking with many others about sharing their cancer diagnosis with their kids, I've learned that it's often harder and more stressful for the afflicted parent than it is for the kids. One woman I know was really stressed about telling her children, worried that they would be worried. They listened, asked a few questions, and went on with their day.

Kids are amazingly resilient. On the first-year anniversary of the end of my chemo treatments, I suggested to my family that we go out to dinner. At dinner, I brought up that we were celebrating a year past chemo. My son said, "Oh, wow, I had forgotten about that."

Taking Action on Talking with Friends and Family, or Not

▶ *Dumb Comments*

Before sharing your cancer news, carefully consider who needs to know and from whom you will get the most support. Oddly, sometimes some of your best friends and family, perhaps thinking that they can be candid, will say the dumbest things. Be prepared, and have a strategy for dealing with the comments.

▶ *Company*

Surround yourself with the people who are most supportive in the way you need support. Feel no guilt in not inviting the company of those who annoy you.

▶ *Social Media*

Consider social media as a way to share your news when and how you want. There are pros and cons, especially in dealing with comments and privacy, but I found it effective and helpful.

▶ *Telling the Kids*

If you are a parent, think through how you will tell your children. Look for guidelines—many are available online. Keep in mind that most kids are more resilient than adults, but your frame of mind and attitude will signal to them how to handle the news.

In summary, here are five actions you can take to talk with friends and family, or not:

1. Be prepared for dumb comments and consider how you will handle them.

2. Keep only the company that is supportive for you at that time.
3. Think about the role social media can play in helping you manage your cancer communications.
4. Appoint a point of contact or lead communicator and let them deal with updates and sharing news.
5. Include your children in your sharing. Kids can be tremendously supportive and resilient.

CHAPTER 10:

Open Yourself to Kindness

I'm not wasting one more minute.
—HODA KOTB, CANCER SURVIVOR
AND TV PERSONALITY

By far, the most surprising thing about going through cancer was the pure and unexpected kindness of people around me. Throughout my life, I've usually been the person who helps take care of others. Need a meal, a hand, a loan, a sounding board? I'm happy to help. As someone who fiercely values her independence and ability to take care of herself, I never really looked to others (except for my husband), asked, or expected too much in the way of help, support, or kindness.

When you are diagnosed with cancer, however, that independence takes a swift and strong blow, and you must depend on a whole host of people—nurses, doctors, family, friends, and strangers—to get through some days. Vulnerability was new to me, and being truly open to kindness was not customary. While driven by desperation, accepting kindness helped me heal physically and emotionally and changed the way I think about showing kindness to others.

As it turns out, there is a whole science behind how kindness helps with healing. Kindness creates a positive emotional state that leads to several health-related benefits, including decreases in anxiety and faster recovery times. According to a recent story in *HuffPost*, "There is even evidence that when a patient listens to less than a minute of compassionate communication from a physician they feel less anxious.... Neuroscience shows that acting with kindness toward others stimulates the reward circuits in our brains, so giving and receiving kindness has a positive effect on physicians and nurses as well."[1]

While kindness may seem like an emotional benefit, it has positive physical implications as well. According to numerous studies, kindness reduces blood pressure and produces anti-inflammatory effects and helps to generate oxytocin, a naturally produced substance known as the "cuddle hormone" or the "love hormone" because it is released when people snuggle up or bond socially. Oxytocin encourages angiogenesis, or the regrowth of blood vessels, which is important for healing wounds. So, in a very real and physical way, kindness heals.

Scientific Links Between Kindness and Healing

In researching kindness and healing, I came across an extensive scientific literature review sponsored by Dignity Health and conducted by the Center for Compassion and Altruism Research and Education (CCARE) at Stanford University. It reveals a large and growing body of scientific evidence that shows kindness holds the power to heal. "We now know that this often overlooked, virtually cost-free remedy has a statistically significant impact on our physical health. For example, the positive effect of kindness is even greater than that of taking aspirin to reduce the risk of a heart attack," according to the study.

This research shows, at the very least, that in healthcare and medicine, kindness shouldn't be viewed as a warm and fuzzy afterthought, something nice to show after the "real" medicine is administered. Rather, "kindness should be viewed as an indispensable part of the healing process."[2]

Interestingly, the concept of kindness is included in the Hippocratic Oath, the oath of ethics typically taken by physicians, for over a century: "I will remember that . . . warmth, sympathy, and understanding may outweigh the surgeon's knife or the chemist's drug."

Indeed, kindness shown by healthcare professionals is powerful. When I had nurses who showed great kindness, it made a big difference in my ability to endure treatment, like my oncology nurses, who knew how to best tap my port for chemo and followed up with me to ensure I was OK.

On the other hand, lack of kindness, or even lack of responsiveness, had a huge, opposite impact. It made me feel like I was wrong or mistaken in what I was feeling and that I was a pain in someone's side rather than being a patient with true medical needs and concerns. That feels awful.

Respect and responsiveness were two forms of kindness that were keys to me changing my chemo treatment. My oral infusion drug, which I was "on" daily for two weeks on and then off for a week, over five months, was administered by a mail-order pharmacy. When I was "on," a representative from the mail-order pharmacy would follow up with me and see how I was tolerating the medication.

As I've mentioned before, at one point in my treatment, my condition turned dire. I started to have extreme gut pain coupled with almost nonstop diarrhea, food aversions, loss of appetite, and rapid weight loss. The oncologist's office was my first line of contact, and I contacted them four or five times to report my decline. "Those things are to be expected" and "try Imodium" were the responses I was getting.

At a very low point, I received a call from the mail-order pharmacy rep. Headed into a meeting and sitting in my car in a parking lot, I described the same symptoms that I was reporting to my doctor's office. She voiced immediate and serious concern and told me I absolutely should not go on that way. She said that she would call the doctor's office and told me to insist on speaking to the doctor as soon as possible. She was both firm and kind.

Her reaction, filled with concern, caring, and kindness, was a turning point in my treatment. She was absolutely right. I should not have been left to deteriorate to such a condition, and I needed to find strength to assert myself, which I did, and it changed the course of my treatment moving forward for the better.

In talking with many cancer survivors, I've heard stories about kindness being extended to them in many ways—by healthcare providers and through advocacy, food chains, prayers, rides, help with housework, and more. In retrospect, I now often feel ashamed that I didn't reach out more to people I knew who were struggling with illness, especially cancer, and show them more kindness, which can be as simple as a text letting them know that I am keeping them in my prayers.

Mary Kay

In 2003, I was first blessed with breast cancer. I did the six months of chemo and weeks of radiation. I must say, chemo is not for sissies. Yes, I lost all my hair. I usually wore a baseball cap. It screamed, Bald head here! I decided to take advantage of this life gift. I found other people were very kind to a bald-headed cancer lady. I never had to take a number at the deli; people stepped aside so I could go next. Cars stopped and drivers waved to me to cross the street safely. I got a seat at events even when they were crowded. I could go through the express lane with more than twelve items and no one said a word. It was the last time I ever shaved my legs. I was blessed!"

Looking at cancer as a blessing is something I still struggle with, but when I talked to Miss Plank, I could see that she genuinely viewed her condition as a blessing with benefits! It's still amazing to me how many people consider their cancer to be a blessing.

Food as Kindness

When I was a kid and was sick, my Nonnie, my mom's mother, would make a homemade Italian soup called pasta rasa. A chicken-broth soup with rice, combined with egg and cheese, pasta rasa was healing, and you could feel her love in the soup. Nonnie and my mom expressed their loving care and kindness through food, and I tend to do the same. In my family, making food for someone is an act of love.

During chemo treatment, food became a very big problem for me, as it does for most chemo patients. My appetite nosedived, I couldn't hold food in my system, every food tasted off, and the cold neuropathy meant I couldn't eat cold or even cool foods or drinks for several days after chemo. The worst, though, were the food aversions. Almost any food that I ate when going through chemo created an aversion effect, meaning I couldn't stand to even think about it, much less consume it, and constantly had to search for new things that I could tolerate. On top of everything else that you go through in cancer treatment, searching for new, nutritious foods that you can get down adds insult to injury.

That's why when several of my relatives and friends sent me food on a regular basis, I appreciated it more than they will ever know. My mom would just show up bearing a quiche, which I would never make for myself, or with a warm homemade soup. She would bring a variety of healthy snacks to my chemo infusion sessions, which were a welcome departure from the processed crackers and cookies that were offered (but that I never ate).

One of my dearest friends lives in Washington, DC. She would ship all sorts of different frozen meals to feed not just me but the whole family. Her shipments were welcome because I didn't have to prepare dinner, which made me nauseous, and she sent things that enabled me to avoid the food aversions. Another friend, a woman whom I had not known for very long but had met at our club swimming pool, kept track of my infusion dates and then prepared and delivered entire meals on the days that I had chemo infusions. Her meals were different and delicious and again fed the whole family. Another dear friend sent me a gratitude journal with a woman on the cover whose image was created by dozens of butterflies. I still use that journal today!

At first, letting someone feed me and my family made me feel extremely vulnerable, almost embarrassed, like I was unable to care for my family. But my friends fed us with such love, along with great food, that I stopped feeling incapable and just appreciated pure kindness. These friends are busy women, working and taking care of their own families, yet they found the time and made the efforts to take care of me and my family. I am eternally grateful.

Other survivors I have talked with have shared similar feelings of being so grateful for the kindness and at the same time humbled almost to the point of embarrassment by the need for help and the abundance of help received.

Stacy

....

I am still humbled by the outpouring of support that we received from family, friends, colleagues, even strangers! There were times during the whole ordeal when I almost felt embarrassed. How could I thank everyone enough? Did we seem grateful enough? The support was vast. From the wraparound support provided by the Valerie Center to fundraisers, gifts, community support, messages, thoughts. I can't even begin to list them all.

Kindness from Oncology Nurses

Oncology nurses, in general, seem to be especially kind and understanding. The nurse who was assigned to work with me on infusions quickly came to know me and what my body would tolerate and what it wouldn't. She was gentle and took extra care when accessing my port with the infusion needle. Knowing that I would have the same nurse and that she would be kind and gentle made trips to the chemo infusion center easier.

At the end of my last chemo treatment, my kind oncology nurse approached me with something I didn't immediately recognize. She handed me what looked like sleigh bells, a group of about six bells, all roped together with a handle. When I saw what she was holding, I remembered seeing pictures and videos of cancer survivors ringing the bells to herald the end of treatment. While I had someone with me for almost every treatment, that day I didn't, and I'm glad. Because when the nurse handed me the bells, I rang them and cried as hard as I've ever cried. It was like the months of stress and treatments were pouring out of my body and soul, in tears.

In retrospect, and after interacting with other cancer patients, ringing the cancer bells seems like it happened in another life. Perhaps it did. At least I had the chance to ring them.

Mary Kay

....

In a Pittsburgh oncologist's office, someone receives their last chemo treatment. A cancer clinic based in Iowa informs their patient they are cancer-free. A children's cancer center near

Seattle, Washington, reads scans telling parents their child
has successfully completed a course of treatment. Participating
in a growing tradition, before leaving for home, these individu-
als ring the "survival bell" that is hanging in the hallway.
Yes, they have something to celebrate! Nurses, aides, and office
staff cheer.

Some survivors are so gracious about cancer treatment and life,
no matter the circumstances. I can't say that I always was, but the
kindness shown to me by my nurses certainly helped.

After the episodes when the chemotherapy regimen wasn't
working well and I demanded different treatment, the clinical nurse
supervisor at the center was assigned to me for scheduling and
questions. She provided her cell phone number and would check
in with me on a regular basis. She was kind and knowledgeable and
helped me navigate the treatments, tests, and second opinions. This
professional kindness was instrumental in improving the state of
my treatment.

Note: At one of my recent oncology checkups, I visited with
both my oncology nurse and the clinical nurse supervisor. According to the supervisor, my requests to have a consistent nurse was a
driving force in assigning consistent nurses to chemo patients on a
regular basis. I thank the nurses for listening and for implementing
patient-centered change!

Taking Action on Opening Yourself to Kindness

▶ *Kindness*
Recognize that kindnesses of many kinds can be healing. Whether
it's from a dear friend or a perfect stranger, a medical professional

or the greeter at the hospital, take in the kindness with a grateful heart. We tend to focus on the negatives, especially when we are sick. Look for the small kindnesses that may be extended to you each and every day and use them as a way to focus your precious energy on positive things.

▶ *Be Kind to Others*

When you are going through cancer treatment and feeling quite miserable and not yourself, it can be easier to be mean and grumpy than to be kind. At least for me it was. I had to remind myself to be kind and, when I did, it had a positive impact on my daily interactions and health.

▶ *Embarrassment*

Don't let pride, embarrassment, or a feeling of needing to repay someone get in the way of accepting kindness. People can be so kind and giving and go out of their way to help you. In my case, I had always been the one who tried to help others, and perhaps my pride got in the way of accepting kind gestures. The kindness can be overwhelming at times, and you might feel like you are not worthy or can't pay back the gestures. Know that true kindness isn't extended with an expectation of return. While I can't pay back those who were so kind to me, I do try to pay it forward through kindness and support of others who may be suffering in some way.

▶ *Oncology Nurses*

Develop a mutually kind relationship with your oncology nurses. If you are being treated for cancer, oncology nurses will be your lifeline. These nurses treat cancer patients all day, every day. It can't be pleasant. While I was guilty of being grumpy during chemo infusions at first, I tried hard to show kindness to the oncology nurses who took such good care of me.

In summary, here are four things you can do to open yourself to kindness:

1. While it's not easy, try to maintain a grateful heart and look for small acts of kindness.
2. Be kind to others.
3. Put your ego aside and accept help and kindness.
4. Be especially kind to your oncology nurses, who are your primary medical caretakers.

CHAPTER 11:

Fake It Till You Make It

Keep your sunny side up,
keep yourself beautiful, indulge yourself.
—BETSEY JOHNSON, CANCER SURVIVOR
AND DESIGNER

A ccording to several studies, including one recently published in *Psychology Today*, there is a scientific connection between looking good and feeling good from a self-esteem perspective. Women, in particular, seem to be susceptible to appearance-based self-esteem.[1] Science has also shown that just the mere act of smiling can lift your mood, lower stress, boost your immune system, and possibly even prolong your life.[2] These are great reasons to smile when you are sick or going through cancer treatment.

Whether you choose to smile or not, or try to look your best or not, just be true to who you are and what makes you feel good. Everyone is different. My way worked for me, and I hope there is advice that works for you, but you make the choice. Looking at different ways of handling a difficult situation can provide helpful options.

When I was introduced to Lisa Lurie by a mutual friend and then started working with her company as a client, I had no idea how close to home her work would strike. Lisa is a cancer survivor and cofounder of Cancer Be Glammed, as well as the woman who so graciously agreed to write the foreword to this book. Lisa and her work were a huge source of inspiration to me when I was undergoing cancer treatment.

There are organizations, including Look Good Feel Better, that have national programs with a focus on helping women who are undergoing cancer treatment feel better by looking better. Look Good Feel Better is a nonmedical public service program that teaches beauty techniques to people with cancer to help them manage the appearance-related side effects of cancer treatment. The program includes lessons on skin and nail care, cosmetics, wigs and turbans, accessories, and styling, helping people with cancer to find some normalcy in a life that is by no means normal.[3]

While it makes perfect sense that looking better or just smiling helps you feel better, it is such a challenge when everything in your mind and body is impacted by cancer and its treatment. My interpretation was to fake it till I made it—from how I dressed and talked to how I worked and exercised. On some days it was an exercise of mind over matter, and on others it was just a good deal of pretending. Sometimes, especially in the privacy of our home, it was not humanly possible to fake or pretend, and cancer treatment just got the best of me. But faking it worked for me a good deal of the time.

In talking with a number of people after my cancer treatment, I learned that most of them never knew what I was dealing with when it was occurring. When I was in the hospital recovering from colectomy surgery, I brought my work notebook and wrote a new business proposal. Another potential new client had contacted me and wanted to talk soon. So I scheduled the call for two days post-op and conducted the call from my hospital bed. I also got that business!

Some people even commented that I looked "so pretty and thin." In fact, I was thin, very thin, having lost 12 percent of my body weight over the course of my treatment. My thinness meant that I had to pin large tucks on both sides of my pants or skirts so that they wouldn't literally fall off my body. I did buy a few pairs of pants that I wasn't swimming in. But I must have had faith that I was going to rebound because I didn't go out and buy a bunch of skinny clothes; I just adapted my wardrobe and broke out the most clingy items I owned.

Maintaining my appearance was actually a big part of what I tried to do, both to maintain my self-esteem and, really, to hide my sickness from the many people I interacted with through work, the kids' school, and social situations. When I needed to go to a meeting or an event, even though it took a great deal of energy, I put on my normal makeup, fixed my hair, and dressed in nice clothes that made me look and feel like I normally did. I couldn't maintain my normal schedule completely and, sadly, had to opt out of school functions and other events, but when I went out, I did my best to look good, or as good I could.

Lisa

....

I am a breast cancer survivor who underwent a double mastectomy, an oophorectomy (removal of the ovaries), and chemotherapy.... I was totally unprepared for the disfiguring physical side effects of surgery and treatment and their emotional blow to my body image and self-esteem. In a very short period of time, I became bald, breast-less, and bloated from steroids. It was soul destroying. When I was battling breast cancer, I found that when I looked better, I felt better, which is why I founded Cancer Be Glammed.

One of the things that posed the biggest problem for me was shoes. One of the side effects of chemo—one that I had never heard about—is blisters. At one point, just a month into my chemo, I took my daughter on a short trip to a lake for a girl's weekend. Golfing with a former client was on the agenda. (Yes, I traveled and tried to act like nothing was wrong.) I put on some cute golf clothes, including shoes, and went and played nine holes. The next day, my feet started to feel sore in spots. I blamed it on the hot sand on the beach at the lake.

By the time I got home, the sore spots had developed into blisters all over my toes and feet. The blisters were so big that my toes looked like they had toes! To enable me just to get around, I had to wear open sandals that would not rub the blisters. It took a few weeks, but the blisters subsided, and I could work my way back into normal shoes, especially for work.

Even at home, I never, not once, stayed in my pajamas all day. It was summer into fall and the weather was warm, so I would put on some comfy golf or yoga clothes. Always one to get up and go, it would have been unusual for me to stay in pajamas normally, so pj's were never appealing to me, even when I had every reason to stay sleepy.

When I did go out to attend events or to business meetings—all of which I did on a weekly basis—I tried my best to act just like I always did. There were times, though, when acting normally proved immensely challenging. When I went into the hospital for the colectomy surgery, it was a Tuesday morning. My daughter's dance recital was on Saturday evening. I was determined to be home to see the recital and told my doctor about my wishes.

As noted previously, while recovering in the hospital, I did everything possible to ensure a quick recovery, ranging from bringing my own chicken soup and using essential oils to getting myself up out of bed and walking as soon as possible. It was hard, but my digestive system kicked in and I was released on Saturday, midday.

That evening, my husband drove me curbside to the front entrance of the recital. I could barely walk and was dealing with a fresh incision and a bloated, sore belly, but I hobbled into the theater and sat in the back row in time to see my daughter dance. It would have been much easier to say I couldn't make it—and everyone would have kindly understood. But I faked it and I made it and got to see the beauty of my daughter's performance.

Just two weeks after the colectomy surgery, I still couldn't drive, so my kind husband dropped me off close to my meeting in the city, so I didn't have to drive or walk very far. The challenges became increasingly difficult with chemo. Chemo for colon cancer targets, well, the colon. Makes sense, right? Well, when you target the colon, the colon gets angry. Angry colons cause things like painful cramping, bloating, and almost nonstop diarrhea, not to mention the resulting hemorrhoids. Twenty trips to the bathroom in an hour was not uncommon for me at one point.

The Challenges of Working through Chemo

For me, carrying on with work worked. In fact, I didn't really give it much thought; working is just a big part of my life. For others, I suspect, whether to continue working can be an important concern if you are undergoing chemotherapy.

The side effects of chemo were most challenging when out in public. At home, my understanding family didn't question or judge my need to use the toilet every fifteen minutes. While my weight loss was quite apparent, I didn't feel the need to camouflage it at home. But in public, it was a different story.

One day, while meeting with a client, I could feel the rumblings. Since I was doing a presentation, I told myself that I had to hold on until it was over. While I thought there was a distinct possibility that I would just shit on my nice client's office chair, my colon cooperated until I ran and escaped to the bathroom. The noise and smell of an angry colon full of chemo drugs is foul, so I waited until everyone in the ladies' room exited before all hell broke loose. Then I exited as quickly as possible, not wanting to be connected to what hopefully no one had to encounter.

On another occasion, I was facilitating a meeting from a podium in front of a group of about thirty people. My gut pain was so bad that I literally held on to the podium while I kept talking just to keep myself from doubling over. The gut pain was so severe that I almost moaned in pain out loud. Focusing as much as I could on the content of the meeting got me through.

Was I stupid to carry on while in so much distress and sometimes pain? Maybe. And maybe it's not for everyone. Several cancer patients with whom I spoke while writing this book preferred to rest in their pajamas for many days. Each person will be different. Do what's best for you.

According to the Cancer Knowledge Network, there is very little published research regarding work patterns, what affects the decision to work, and support from employers during active cancer treatment. The decision and ability to continue working is very personal, with physical and mental health, type and stage of cancer, age, type of work, and finances all part of the consideration set.[4]

Keeping my work routine helped me stay sane and heal. It took my mind off what I was going through and gave me purpose. Fortunately, I didn't seem to experience the "chemo brain" syndrome that so many people talk about. "Chemo brain" is a term that cancer patients and survivors use to describe a sort of cognitive fog that seems to impact memory and other brain functions. Was it because I kept busy and maintained a pretty regular schedule? I can't say for sure, but working helped me.

One other piece of advice that Lisa Lurie gave me was not to take on too much work during chemo, so I'd have the flexibility for self-care and days off, if needed. I did maintain a lighter-than-normal work schedule, but I only took off about three days during my entire cancer ordeal and chemo treatment. In fact, I'd often take my laptop to the chemo infusion center and work away during the four to six hours I'd have to spend there.

Dressing for Success

At Children's Hospital of Pittsburgh, there was a five-year-old girl named Lilli who was being treated for cancerous growths on her optic nerve. Lilli decided to wear a different princess gown to each of her twenty chemotherapy treatments. She may need future treatments, but Lilli seems to be doing well. God bless Lilli and her health. While I am probably too old for princess dresses, I understand where Lilli was coming from, and just looking business casual helped me.

Speaking of the chemo infusion center, that's a place where it's tough to fake how you are feeling. It's still surreal to me that I was one of the many patients—and I do mean many, as in constant full house—being treated for cancer. The way I dealt with it was to treat it like I was going to work.

When I had a chemo infusion day, I'd dress "business casual," something comfortable but nice. My philosophy has always been that you get treated by others at a level that you look and dress. It's why I always try to dress nicely when I travel, and I applied the same logic to medical treatment.

Turns out that most people, understandably so, go to chemo infusion centers in sweats or pajamas. Several of the nurses and aids in the center commented to me on how nice I always looked. For me, I felt less sick when I appeared not sick.

Exercise

Exercise was another activity that I felt strongly about keeping in my life. In fact, there is scientific evidence that exercise is a good practice during chemotherapy treatment. The American Cancer Society recommends that, if possible, cancer patients avoid inactivity and return to normal daily activities as soon as possible following a cancer diagnosis: 150 minutes of moderate-intensity aerobic exercise or seventy-five minutes of vigorous-intensity exercise per week, including strength-building exercises at least two days per week.[5]

Inactivity is not for me, though maintaining anything even close to my normal workout routine was not possible. After my colectomy surgery, I was forced to curtail lifting weights, doing aerobics, practicing yoga, and swinging a golf club—pretty much everything I did. Immediately post-surgery, I remember coming home and only being allowed to walk the steps in my house once a day. What was left? Walking. So I substituted walking for almost all my other activities. At first, I could only walk one lap around the outside of my house. After a few days, I ventured into the lower part of our yard and made the laps much longer.

Then I started to walk the cart path at a golf course very near to our house. Starting very early, before golfers would be on the course, I walked a short part of the course. Then I added on another half mile, then another mile, and another. My daily walk turned into a three-mile hike, up and down hills at the golf course.

The walk, and the beauty and peacefulness of nature on the golf course, was refreshing and healing. Along with my husband and son, I started to walk the golf course and take my wedge and putter so I could chip and putt, though I was still unable to fully swing a driver or iron.

I maintained this exercise schedule through the start of chemo. But then chemo made me very tired, and my gut was in serious pain. When I'd walk down hills at the golf course, I'd moan out loud in pain as my feet moved me forward and down the hill. The gut pain was relentless and became too much. Even the walking had to stop for a period of a month or so while my body railed against the chemo and left me just enough energy to work and do the bare minimum to take care of my family.

As soon as I could muster the strength, I started walking again. Both the physical benefits—building stamina, fresh air, improved muscle tone—and the mental benefits—a clear mind, taking in nature, and distraction—all had a positive effect on my mind and body.

Travel

Traveling is one of the best ways I have found to expand my horizons, learn how to troubleshoot, appreciate differences, and distract my mind. For many years, I was a road warrior for work, making dozens of work trips every year and racking up the highest levels of frequent-flier miles. Even with so many travel experiences, I always learned something new and often had to solve some problem I had never encountered previously. And even though I was often on the road for work, my family and I traveled extensively for pleasure, always learning, enjoying new things, and problem-solving together. If you are a traveler at heart, being true to your "travel bug," even during cancer, could be an important part of your healing.

My business still requires me to travel by air to meet on site with clients or to attend conferences and events, though COVID-19 has certainly restricted travel. Given how my body was reacting to chemo, traveling even by car became challenging. With long days, getting through airports, walking in big cities, and working in groups, it takes a lot of energy to travel even on a good day. When your energy and immune systems are depleted, you have digestive distress, you need frequent access to a bathroom, and you are dealing with blisters the size of quarters, it's even more challenging. Still, I traveled. Not as much as I might normally, but I did it.

On one trip in particular, I was early on in my chemo treatment, and I didn't yet realize how fatiguing travel would be. Per my usual when traveling, I was up way before dawn and on the first flight out to Chicago. My schedule took me to several meetings and, because I enjoy walking, I walked to and from my appointments in the city.

When I was on the plane on the way home that same night, the fatigue started to settle in. By the time I arrived in the Pittsburgh airport, I thought I might need a wheelchair to get me from the plane to my car. Not one to take my time much when in airports, I slowly walked the length of the airport corridor, determined to make it on my own volition. And I did. Which reminds me: be kind in airports— and everywhere for that matter; you never know what battle someone traveling beside you is fighting.

Some people might ask why I didn't just rest and let my body heal? For me, healing has a lot to do with being me and not a compromised version of myself, so I tried to do what I normally did. In a sense, I was faking it, because I didn't feel myself. On the other hand, I was being true to who I am. Everyone is different, and to each her own. My advice is to be true to yourself and who you were before cancer to understand how you can best heal during cancer.

The other morning, at the gym, I thought about how when I was in chemo treatment, I could not even lift ten pounds. Now, I can exercise on a regular schedule and do pretty much anything I want. Yoga, lifting weights, and playing golf are all part of my life again. In fact, I am lifting more weight and have a better golf game than prior to cancer!

Regular CT scans, blood work, and oncology appointments serve to remind me that I am still in recovery. Other than those unnerving times when I must focus on health surveillance, I go on with my life and pretend that I am just the normal me.

Taking Action on Faking It till You Make It

▶ *Dress the Part*

Dress for cancer treatment in a way that makes you feel good. Whether it's business casual, princess dresses, or something in between, an outside appearance that accentuates your best has an amazing power to make you feel better.

▶ *Keep Moving*

Energy begets energy. You may not feel like it, but getting the blood flowing with some light exercise can have a healing impact on your mind and body. Think about your exercise routine prior to treatment, and try to maintain as many parts of it as possible. I am an advocate for walking in and of itself, as exercise and as a complement to a broader exercise regime. Both the physical and mental dimensions of walking, especially if you walk somewhere where you can take in nature, are healing.

▶ *Working*

You'll work it out—if you are working, see how your work can play a positive role in your healing. Working can take your mind off your woes and enable you to feel productive. Having the option to lighten a full-time workload is helpful, as is having the option to rest on days that you need it. Don't feel pressured to know at the beginning how you'll work during the duration of your treatment. Sometimes you have to take it day by day.

▶ *Travel*

If travel is normally an enjoyable part of your life for business or pleasure, find a way to continue traveling. It may require special arrangements, but if travel feeds your soul, it can and should still be a part of your life and can contribute to normalcy and healing.

▶ *Try to Be You*

Faking it, to me, was all about trying to be the real me when, in reality, I was a compromised and different version of myself during cancer treatment. Everyone is different. Be who you are, and try to not let the circumstances of cancer treatment turn you into someone you aren't or don't want to be.

In summary, here are five things you can do to fake it till you make it:

1. Dress the part.
2. Keep moving.
3. Work it out—try to maintain some sort of work schedule.
4. Travel.
5. Try to be you.

CHAPTER 12:

Watch for Miracles

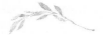

A huge part of my success as an athlete was that I had the mental game. To get through the toughest moments of treatment, I relied on goal setting and keeping that positive mentality.
—SHANNON MILLER, CANCER SURVIVOR
AND FORMER OLYMPIC GYMNAST

Being told you have cancer has a way of putting a damper on things. It can be hard to see life's everyday magic, and it's easy to focus on the pain, suffering, and fear. In the days immediately after my colonoscopy, without even having full confirmation, I spent most of the time feeling numb and crying.

The feeling was one of being sucker punched, living in a state of disbelief of what had just happened and having no idea of what the future held. There I was, leading basically the same life as I had been the day before, but my outlook had flipped from happy and relatively carefree to miserably unhappy and scared out of my mind.

In that state of mind, my grasp on positivity was lost, and that was hard to shake amid the chaos of a cancer journey. A shocking diagnosis is often followed by a dizzying number of calls with doctors' offices, hospitals, and insurance carriers; doctor's appointments and tests; and constant thought about your condition. The amount of work I needed to do to navigate the healthcare system could have been a full-time job. I'm not sure how people who don't have job flexibility are able to manage what amounts to a third shift but has to happen during daytime business hours.

During this time, many of the routine things in my life had to be changed or were taken away from me. The one cup of hot black coffee that I enjoyed every morning began to taste terrible and make me nauseous. The simple act of making my daughter's lunch in the morning became almost unbearable because touching cold things with my hands, like lettuce for a salad, made my fingers sting and burn from the cold neuropathy. So many small actions that I had taken for granted during the day were now painful or simply not doable.

While I had been practicing yoga for years, it was almost impossible to calm and clear my mind or to see the everyday beauty and miracles in life that I so often had seen before. Even sleep became difficult as thoughts raced both day and night. It's probably not a surprise to learn that my feelings and attitudes were quite normal. According to the National Cancer Institute, just as cancer affects your physical health, it can bring up a wide range of feelings you're not used to dealing with. Stress, anxiety, guilt, and feelings of being overwhelmed are all common emotions and reactions to a cancer diagnosis.[1]

The National Cancer Institute has some helpful information for dealing with these complex emotions on topics including expressing your feelings, being active, helping yourself relax, choosing when you talk about your cancer, ways to remain in control, and, one I especially like, looking for positives. When dealing with cancer, I came to see any positive as a miracle.

Recently, *Psychology Today* tackled this topic in an article titled "Do You Believe in Miracles? Turning to Divine Intervention When Facing Serious Medical Illness." As it turns out, believing in miracles is somewhat common. Holding these beliefs is not limited to certain age groups, nor is it restricted to certain religious denominations or a religious affiliation.

According to the article, "Discovering that you or a loved one is seriously medically ill can be devastating, particularly if the prognosis is poor. Among the various responses to this type of news, such as experiencing disbelief, anguish, and worry, many people turn to spiritual support—including the hope for a miracle."

In my experience, I didn't hear doctors refer to miracles, but apparently even physicians believe in miracles. In a national poll of 1,100 physicians from different religious faiths, the physicians were asked whether they believed in miracles. "Seventy-four percent believed miracles had occurred in the past and 73 percent held the belief that miracles occur today."[2]

Sometimes miracles presented themselves as something that just went right in the midst of all hell breaking loose. When I underwent my first CT scan to take a look at the extent of potential cancer beyond the polyp in my colon, the doctors spotted a nodule in my left breast. That made me shit a brick and sent me into a tailspin to get an urgent diagnostic mammogram. The mammogram showed the nodule, but it looked like some sort of calcification, not cancer. While I can't ever say that in my past *not* having breast cancer after being diagnosed with colon cancer would top my list of miracles, it certainly did.

Then there were the everyday miracles. Every morning when I woke up, I had a newfound appreciation for life. With so many things that can possibly go wrong, just waking up and breathing is miraculous. Each morning, I'd say the words "thank you" when each of my feet hit the floor, and then I'd continue with the thanks as I navigated each step down to the kitchen. Throughout the day, "thank you" has become a mantra when recognizing these small but powerful miracles, whether it's the bright blue color of the sky on a clear day or the smell of cookies baking in the oven.

Encountering so many sick people like never before in hospitals and treatment centers, I found it miraculous that my condition was detected relatively early and that my condition, while challenging, was much better than many others. Walking into a cancer treatment center is sad and sickening. Walking out is sad and humbling. Ringing the cancer bells and walking out healthy is a miracle.

Brandie

At my very first mammogram at the young age of forty, I was diagnosed with Stage IV breast cancer. I was a mother of four beautiful children and had a wonderful husband and family. I grieved for them more than anything. I knew I could only control how I reacted to the situation and that I had to be strong. I put my faith in God, praying every day, sometimes all day. I felt the miracles happening. My oncologist told me she could see the difference faith made in my healing, and even though she was of a different faith, she prayed for me as well. I am three and a half years out now, in complete remission, closer to God, and grateful for everything.

Once I was through treatment, miracles also took the form of a restoration of normalcy that I had previously taken for granted, perhaps: being able to move without pain, appreciating the details of nature while on a walk, packing a lunch without thinking twice, lifting more than ten pounds, and making progress at the gym.

Coffee never tasted so good as when the chemo was out of my system, my taste buds had healed, and I could sit with my cats in the morning, feeling normal. Being able to eat Thanksgiving dinner and really taste turkey, gravy, and mashed potatoes is one of my best post-chemo memories.

Some people think of miracles as divine intervention. My version of miracles certainly includes the power of God to create healing, show us the beauty of nature, and provide clues to the path that best suits us. Quite a few people I have encountered say things like "I am putting everything in God's hands," sometimes with the idea that God will take care of everything and they don't have to do anything. However, miracles, in my opinion, are usually the combination of divine intervention and human action working together. I asked God to show me the path to miracles, but I had to make it happen.

Anna

Even when faced with the direst of situations, you can always encounter uplifting and encouraging moments, as long as you are open to experiencing them. I was told by my doctors that I had two separate Stage IV metastatic cancers ravaging my body at the same time, which in essence meant that any chance of survival would require a miracle. Not being sure if one was just going to drop in my lap, I decided to create one (or more) myself. My treatments consisted of two phases separated by a month's break. During that break, I planned a trip to Maui, a place that was particularly dear to my heart. My daughter accompanied me, and we experienced the most phenomenal whale-watching encounter. The whales swam and frolicked so close to our boat that we could see the barnacles attached to their fins as well as scratches on their bodies. Being able to witness the beauty of these magnificent creatures so close was nothing short of a miracle. The greater miracle, however, was how the encounter made me forget about being sick, lifted my spirits, and filled my soul with optimism and encouragement that my fight to recover was worth the grueling effort. We are surrounded by miracles; we just have to know where to look.

Never having gone through surgery prior to my cancer journey, I can now say that how a human body handles and heals from surgery is miraculous. To think that a human body can be opened up, parts can be taken out, other parts can be sewn back together, and you can get up a few days later and walk away is amazing and nothing short of a miracle to me.

After my surgery and then post-chemo, my body was certainly weakened, barely able to lift a ten-pound weight, which I had done regularly prior. Step by step, determined to get back into good physical shape, I began lifting weights again. It took a year, but I have worked my way back and now use 17.5-pound dumbbells for my work out. Miracle.

When faced with a problem, a spat with someone, or a challenge, in my mind I say, *This is nothing compared to cancer. If I can overcome cancer, I can do this, whatever it is.* My mindset has become even stronger and more positive, which I consider to be an ongoing series of miracles.

Ever since the chemo treatments ended, I've undergone a series of surveillance tests, including blood work and a CT scan. All results have been, as I've expected, normal. No sign of cancer. That's a serious miracle.

Susan

....

I learned to see the good and realized how grateful I am for all my experiences that have led me to this point—positive and negative—and all those that will be.

Taking Action on Watching for Miracles

▶ *Everyday Miracles*

First, I've tried to reground myself by recognizing that each and every facet of life is a miracle. You woke up this morning? Miracle. You are breathing? Miracle. Your family has enough food to eat? Miracle. A butterfly landed on a flower in my yard, enabling me to take a look at its beautiful and fragile wings? Miracle. Especially when you are facing cancer, every part of your life can produce miracles, if you look for and recognize them.

▶ *Action*

If you've read enough of this book, you'll see that I'm big on taking action. If you do nothing, nothing will change. Action begets miracles. While miracles are not nearly as neat and predictable as you or I might like them to be, moving ahead in some ways opens new possibilities that can lead to new, miraculous solutions.

▶ *Trust God*

As firm believer in a God that wants good for us, it helped me to take comfort in trusting in that goodness. No matter your beliefs, I advocate for trusting in goodness.

▶ *Stay in Shape*

Help your body produce miracles by taking care of yourself physically and mentally.

▶ *Take, and Celebrate, Little Wins*

Every little health win matters and is a reason to celebrate when you are working your way through cancer. Don't wait for the end of treatment or a major breakthrough. Acknowledge each step along the way.

▶ *Move Forward*

Focusing on happy plans for the future, whether a trip, a special family celebration, or just a good meal, kept me focused on the end goal, not the current circumstances.

▶ *Gratitude, Again*

An ongoing theme throughout my experience and in this book, gratitude has been a key tool in helping me transition from cancer patient to cancer survivor.

In summary, here are seven things you can do to look for miracles:

1. Don't take anything for granted. See every little thing as a miracle.
2. Take action on your own behalf to create your own miracles.
3. Look to God, and help her do her work.
4. Stay in shape, physically and mentally.
5. Recognize health progress.
6. Move forward.
7. See the good and be grateful.

CHAPTER 13:

You Are Stronger
Than You Know

Women are like teabags. We don't know our
true strength until we are in hot water.
—ELEANOR ROOSEVELT

W hen you are told you have cancer, no matter how strong you were previously, it's a blow that's extremely difficult to take. According to WebMD, and perhaps according to just about anyone, "cancer" may be the most frightening word in medicine. The initial shock gives way to a realization of the tremendous physical, emotional, and spiritual challenges that lie ahead.[1] In short, life changes in the flip of a switch when you are told you have cancer, and you feel vulnerable, out of control, and as if any strength you possessed has left you.

Amazingly, though, and consistently throughout all my discussions and interactions with other cancer patients, being stronger than they knew was a prevailing theme. You don't know how you'll make it through, but somehow you find the strength and you do.

In my experience, strength takes a variety of forms. First there is the mental strength to get through the shock of diagnosis and to keep yourself together enough to navigate and cope. Then there is physical strength, which is compromised and which dwindles during a time of intense changes to your body. When you go about your daily life, you rarely look at the basics of living as something that requires strength; you just do it. With cancer, just putting one foot in front of another each day requires immense strength.

"Live! Don't wait for permission to live. Just because you have cancer does not mean that your life is over," insists Kris Carr, author of *Crazy Sexy Cancer Tips*. "Start living. It's that simple."[2] It sounds simple, and indeed it's true. But when diagnosed with cancer, just living requires you to tap into unknown strength.

Sylvia

....

I think the most surprising thing I learned during my arduous journey with two cancers simultaneously was strength. I heard someone say, "We never know how strong we are until being strong is the only choice we have." I had that quote on a chalkboard in my kitchen that I read with every surgery, MRI, CT scan, chemo treatment, and radiation. It set the stage for me, as I left my home to embark on each of these! I was stronger than ever imaginable!

What's especially hard is knowing that cancer is at the least a short-term, painful, and stressful journey, and that it possibly can bring a lifetime of health challenges and treatment. When I was diagnosed, it was hard to think about anything but cancer, and I've heard others say the same. Thinking about or trying to make plans makes you realize how uncertain and unpredictable the future is.

My family likes to travel, and we are usually planning a family trip for some time in the future. Several times during chemo treatment, we were invited to join friends on trips—one to Abu Dhabi and Dubai to watch a Formula One race, something we had never done before. Before the chemo really started to make me sick, we looked into flights and talked about an itinerary. Over a short time, the chemo really started to affect me, and it became clear that my body could barely handle daily life and there would be no such trip in my immediate future. I wanted to pretend like I would be fine and that by the time the trip came along, I'd be ready to roll. That kind of thinking usually kept me going. But my physical condition was rapidly deteriorating, and I knew that thirteen hours on a plane and a week full of activity in a foreign country was a plan that not even I could pull off.

Much to my dismay, we declined going on the trip. At that moment, it felt like I might never go on another trip again. But once chemo was over, my physical strength grew. I started traveling again, first for business, and then, by March, we were able to make a trip to Jamaica.

Living with uncertainty is challenging. One of the ways that I began to cope with it was to ask God for signs. In my heart, I knew everything would work out in time, so I asked God to show me my path with signs. Those signs somehow gave me strength and courage to continue going, knowing that I was on the right path.

Susan

....

I learned I handle fear and agony with quiet grace and unfailing faith. I learned I'm more resilient than I already knew I was and able to navigate uncertainty with a silent knowing that God is guiding my steps.

My sister gave me a cross printed with the saying "Let your faith be bigger than your fear." It hangs on a frequently used cabinet in my kitchen, and I read it many times a day. There were days when I would look at it, read it, and cry. The tears were sometimes of sadness and sometimes of joy, as the saying hit home for me. Reading and keeping handy the most meaningful inspirational sayings helped focus my mind in a positive direction.

Another motivator for me was seeing so many sick people in the chemo infusion center. It was always full, every day. Reading statistics does not tell the story or show the human side of the disease. After spending hours and hours in the infusion center, it seemed to me that almost everyone in there had it worse than me. They were mostly older, thin, worn down, and sick looking. Seeing my fellow cancer patients in that setting inspired my strength, as my condition seemed to pale in comparison.

Praying for all my fellow infusion mates was an effective way for me to be helpful and find strength, even in my weakened condition. Everyone in that infusion center was suffering in some way, whether a patient or someone who accompanied that patient. Simple acts of kindness, like offering a snack or just a smile, helped others and helped me realize that there is strength in the simplest of actions.

There was one young man, in his twenties, whom I encountered in the chemo infusion center. He was seated in the same pod for several of his treatments. Seeing him, thin but resolute, gave me strength. Having cancer in your fifties is crappy, but to be that young and have cancer is almost incomprehensible and unfair.

When dealing with cancer, I was stronger than I knew. But needing to deal with a cancer diagnosis for a child must be almost as hard as it can get, requiring more strength than ever imaginable. To all of those who have had to deal with such circumstances, my heart goes out to you, and I keep you in my prayers.

Stacy
....

People would say to me all the time, "I don't know how you do it. I would be a ball of misery on the floor." And I would say, "I don't have a choice. What else can I do? I have two other children in addition to my sick child, and if I am not positive, productive, and hopeful, what does it mean for them?" Again, I don't hold it against any of these friends. They just don't know. I probably thought the same things when I was in their shoes. But what I wish anyone just starting this journey would realize is that you do have the strength. You just don't know it. You wouldn't be on the floor in a puddle of sadness. You would be doing the same thing that I am doing.

If you or a loved one are experiencing cancer, keep going. You can do it. It can get better. In retrospect, it's easier to see that cancer and its treatment doesn't last forever. While making plans may need to be shelved for a time, life gradually returns.

During my three weeks of chemo break, I started to bounce back and realized that how I came to feel during chemo treatment would not be a new normal. I could recover. There was light at the end of the tunnel.

The nurses who were assigned to me for overall care and for chemo treatments made all the difference in the world. The consistency and familiarity, coupled with their care and kindness, promoted healing and recovery much more than there was previously.

Finally, in early November, after four torturous months, I had my last infusion. Hoping the chemo off-ramp would be gentle was a pipe dream. I had lost over 12 percent of my body weight. My appetite and energy were low, and my neuropathy lingered. After about a month, I could feel some significant, positive changes. My appetite was returning. I felt like working out. I started to cook, not bothered by smells or food aversions.

As life returns, celebrate every little victory. Chemo is over—take the day off and do something you love. Feeling a bit more energetic—take a longer walk or get a massage. A clear scan—have a special dinner. Focus as much as possible on any positive news or change and mark it. The celebration creates strength around good news and positive movement.

At one year post-chemo, surveillance tests were conducted. A CT scan and blood work were ordered in advance of an oncologist appointment. My instincts and heart told me that I was fine, but going to the hospital to get tests that are cancer-related can be disconcerting. My attitude was mostly positive. Because I find strength in taking action and control, I asked to be notified as soon as my test results were ready.

When the results were available, I went directly to medical records at the hospital, got my own copy, and read them. (Yes, I've learned how to read the technicalities of CT scans and blood work reports.) That way, I had confirmation that everything was fine, which it was, and I did not have to wait a week for my oncologist to tell me that everything was fine. When the day of my oncologist appointment arrived, I could go to it knowing with confidence that all was well.

What I have realized is that the biggest factor in my treatment and healing was me. When my attitude, positivity, and courage to speak up for myself waned, so did my physical condition. That's not to say that attitude, positivity, and self-advocacy alone can heal cancer, but they play a prominent role, alongside the medical dimensions of treatment. And those are the things that are really under your control, and feeling in control with cancer, as much as humanly possible, is a major advantage.

Taking Action on Being Stronger Than You Know

▶ *Seek Out Motivational Reading*

Read and keep motivational and inspirational quotes and sayings close by so you can see them often. Pause, take in the message, and try to carry it with you throughout your day.

▶ *Keep Living*

Try to see putting one foot in front of the other as enough. Just one step and then another.

▶ *Stay Open*

Don't stay put in your house and hunker down unless your immune system is too compromised. Stay open to the world, its beauty, and its distractions.

▶ *Think of Others*

In the cancer world, there are so many others who have it harder than you do at any given time. If they can do it, you have the strength too.

▶ *Be Helpful*

Thinking of others when you are sick is hard, but it will remind you that you can be helpful, even in a weakened condition. Take strength in being helpful.

▶ *Pray*

Pray, if you are so inclined, for your fellow patients and for your own healing.

▶ *Get Your Test Results*

Pick up your own test results from medical records or the medical facility, and get a sense for the results. If they are fine, put your mind at ease. If there are issues, call the doctor's office and ask them to call you as soon as possible to discuss. Don't wait days or weeks with a worried mind to find out the results of a test.

▶ *Celebrate*

Celebrate every bit of positive news in whatever way makes you happiest—take the afternoon off, go golfing (like I do), treat yourself to a special dinner, see a concert—whatever helps you mark the good news and remember that things can change.

In summary, here are eight things you can do to take action on staying strong:

1. Use inspirational quotes or sayings.
2. Keep living.
3. Stay open.
4. Think of others.
5. Be helpful to others.
6. Pray.
7. Get your own test results.
8. Celebrate every little bit of good news.

Epilogue

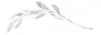

For six months, while I posted on Facebook about family, work, and fun; traveled to client meetings; and shaped a public persona of normalcy, I was secretly battling a cancer diagnosis and undergoing chemotherapy treatments. Some observant people commented that I looked thin in my pictures, with the implication that something must be wrong. I confirmed nothing. Some people commented that I must be working out extra hard to stay so thin and thought I looked great. I said, "Thank you." Except for a handful of my closest family and friends, I didn't divulge my secret. It was too painful, and somehow admitting the truth would make it more real. Maybe it wouldn't be so real if I just went about my life.

During my diagnosis and treatment, I began to seek divine guidance and visited the chapel where I attended college and was later married. The chapel was less than a mile from our house and had always been a place of comfort, quiet, and prayer for me. On one occasion, when I was there praying quietly, for some reason I looked up. When I looked up I noticed that a large hanging pendant light was swaying ever so slightly.

How odd.

As I watched the light move back and forth, my eye was drawn from the light to the large rosette stained-glass window—one of two in the chapel. Within the design of the rosette, there were swirls that looked like butterflies. I was floored. All the times that I had been to the chapel, including for my own wedding, and I had never noticed the similarities to butterflies. God was speaking directly to me and telling me I was on the right path, however difficult.

I still feel like I am the healthiest person I know. Writing this book was hard because every time I sat down to write, it brought me back to a place that seemed like an alternate universe or a bad dream. Did I really have cancer? Even though I just completed my year after chemo scans and tests, in some ways it feels like it was never really me. Then I look at the surgical scar on my lower abdomen, the scar from the port that was inserted into the right side of my chest wall, and I see so many reminders that I realize it was indeed me.

Many fellow survivors say that getting cancer was a blessing and that they have learned and gained so much on their cancer journey. Cancer certainly presents opportunities to learn more than you can in a four-year college education. It also helps you gain perspective on what really matters in life—whatever that is to each individual person. When everything is at risk, perspective comes quickly. Calling cancer a blessing is still a struggle for me. It's a path that God has chosen for me, for some reason, and one that God led me through. The question of "Why this path?" is still unanswered.

Learning to trust my instincts and be my own health advocate has been invaluable, and perhaps someone reading this book will become better prepared to be their own advocate or an advocate for a loved one. And I never did call my surgeon of choice on his cell phone, but I took advantage of the back-office nurse line, where the nurses were helpful in answering questions.

Today, I am on a train, traveling to New York with my son for a conference. In some ways, life just goes on and you keep working, living. In other ways, I find it's not business as usual. My level of gratitude for being able to spend time with my son, on this particular trip, and for my family, each day, is deeper than ever before.

There was a quote on a LinkedIn post that I read today that said, "Stories help others. Share yours." While talking recently to a friend who had been diagnosed with breast cancer and just underwent a bilateral mastectomy, she said she had read my published story "Butterflies in My Stomach." She went on to say that she and her family had taken several of the actions that I recommended and that they helped her. It is my hope that by sharing my story, others will find the help they need on their cancer journey.

"Butterflies In My Stomach"

Medium, June 5, 2018

I never really paid that much attention to news coming out of the American Cancer Society, but today I did. New guidelines recommend that US adults start colon cancer screening earlier, at age forty-five, instead of fifty. I agree wholeheartedly. I'm a fairly private person, not one to broadly share deeply personal experiences, but I feel the need to speak out and share. Here's why:

I am the healthiest person I know—the one in a million who exercises every day, eats from the local farmer's market, wakes up every day feeling energized, and rarely gets a cold. That's why, just a month ago, when I went for my first routine colonoscopy, I assumed it was just a one-day pain in the butt, literally. Coming out of the post-procedure fog of the propofol, however, I remember the doctor saying words like "cancerous polyp," "CT scan," and "when you talk to the surgeon." In an instant, the healthy bubble I lived in popped—or more like exploded.

While I have experienced many things and am a calm, competent professional, none of that prepared me for the health-scare-induced whirlwind of the past few weeks, where I've spent more time in hospitals and doctors' offices than at a full-time job. Someone likened it to opening the hood of a vintage car (thanks, I'm not *that* old)—you identify something that is causing it not to run right but, in the process, discover other parts that need fixing. So it went with me.

There was, indeed, an asymptomatic but large cancerous polyp. It was removed. Relief. The only way to know how far it reached was to do blood work (which came back clear) and a CT scan, which did not indicate spreading but did show a nodule in my left lung. Mild panic. A second CT scan with a focus on the lung showed a nodule in my left breast. Hard to breathe. The diagnostic mammogram indicated benign calcium in my breast but thought the nodule may be in my liver. Going to puke. After two nerve-wracking, nail-biting weeks of testing, the nodules were determined to be clear. Lost eight pounds. In the meantime, my husband and I were simultaneously talking to surgeons about the recommended course of treatment for the polyp site, which turned out to be major abdominal surgery. What??? Whose life is this???

That surgery, a colectomy, where about ten inches of my sigmoid colon and associated lymph nodes were removed, took place one week ago. I went from doing yoga in the preoperative holding area to temporarily being unable to eat, pee, or move on my own postoperatively. Fortunately, I had a fantastic surgical team, led by Dr. Kenneth Lee, at UPMC's Presbyterian Hospital in Pittsburgh, who was committed to medical excellence as well as to getting me home for my daughter's recital. I can't say enough about professional and compassionate and terrific nursing care on the tenth floor of Montefiore hospitals. Equally important, my husband was by my side every step of the way, and my mom, kids, sister, and friends rallied around me. I was discharged four days after the surgery, in time to see my daughter's dance recital. I sit here today, one week post-op, sharing my experiences with you. God is good.

I learned a few lessons along the way that I thought would be of interest.

1. Get a second medical opinion and compare. Prepare to ask tough questions, and find the best doctor for you. The doctor's staff and office make a huge difference. You can only know which doctors, staff, and hospital system is right for you if you have something to compare them to. I asked and my surgeon gave me his cell phone number. The office staff got back to me fast. That access and urgency was important to me. Know what's important to you and compare; don't settle.

2. Be aware of opioids and ask about options. Opioids and narcotics are routinely used during and after surgery. Given the opioid epidemic in this country, I wanted to stay away from anything that could be addictive. I talked extensively with anesthesiology professionals and learned my options. I chose to be part of an accelerated recovery program that reduced the use of opioids and narcotics. In the week since my surgery, I've used only Tylenol and Advil for pain management. Ask and know your options about anesthesiology and pain management.

3. Inconvenient kindness is healing. A dear girlfriend drove four hours each way to visit me for an hour and to deliver groceries to my house. A friend who is a priest, and happens to help run St. Vincent College, made a special trip, out of his way and unasked, to administer anointing of the sick to me in the hospital. My husband, mom, and sister were at the hospital with me to check in at 5:00 a.m. and stayed, and stayed and stayed. All of these people had other things to do, and it was not convenient to do what they did. That inconvenient kindness touched my heart and soul and accelerated my healing. I need to do more of it for others.

4. Nutrition and sleep are critical to recovery but hard to come by in a hospital. My post-op clear-liquid diet consisted of basically sugar water—besides Ensure Clear and bouillon broth, I was given Snack Pack Jell-O, sherbet, lemonade, grape juice, apple juice, and cranberry juice. (Tip 1: I made my own soup and brought it with me.) There has to be a better and more scientific nutritional approach to postoperative recovery. With the unusually loud beeps of the hallway heart monitor screens, it was impossible for me to sleep. I slept about twelve nonconsecutive hours in three nights. There has to be a way to create a more restful recovery environment. (Tip 2: the last night I got smart and asked for melatonin, which did help.)

5. Ask and look for signs. I made a deal with God—show me butterflies as my guides, and I will follow. Guess what, butterflies showed up. In the examination room of the ob-gyn's office where I was for my post-CT breast exam, there was a random picture of a butterfly taped to the wall. When I had my first surgical appointment, an OR nurse was in the coffee line with me and she had butterflies on her surgical cap. Unbelievably, there were many others. Those signs lit my path and helped guide decisions.

Now I'm working on recovery—walking, but no yoga or golf in the short term; getting back to work (I was able to send out a proposal and do a new business call from the hospital!); and enjoying time with my loving family, who is taking good care of me. I await final pathology results, but I know in my heart that everything will be OK.

If you are forty-five, go get that colonoscopy, even if you are the healthiest person you know.

Notes

Introduction

1. "Colorectal cancer statistics," American Institute for Cancer Research, https://www.wcrf.org/dietandcancer/colorectal-cancer-statistics/.
2. "When Should You Start Getting Screened for Colorectal Cancer?," American Cancer Society, February 4, 2021, https://www.cancer.org/latest-news/american-cancer-society-updates-colorectal-cancer-screening-guideline.html.

Chapter 2

1. Shelley Levitt, "Go With Your Gut: The Science of Instinct," Success, October 27, 2016, https://www.success.com/go-with-your-gut-the-science-of-instinct/.
2. Leo Carver, "How to Recognize Signs From the Universe," Chopra, August 7, 2019, https://chopra.com/articles/how-to-recognize-signs-from-the-universe.

Chapter 3

1. Jane Weaver, "More people search for health online," NBC News, July 16, 2003, https://www.nbcnews.com/id/wbna3077086.

2. Megan Brenan, "Nurses Again Outpace Other Professions for Honesty, Ethics," Gallup, December 20, 2018, https://news .gallup.com/poll/245597/nurses-again-outpace-professions -honesty-ethics.aspx.

3. "What is the U.S. Opioid Epidemic?," U.S. Department of Health and Human Services, last reviewed February 19, 2021, https:// www.hhs.gov/opioids/about-the-epidemic/index.html.

4. Jennifer M. Hah, MD, MS, et al., "Chronic Opioid Use After Surgery: Implications for Perioperative Management in the Face of the Opioid Epidemic," *Anesthesia & Analgesia* 125 no. 5 (November 2017), doi.org/10.1213/ANE.0000000000002458.

5. "Information for Health Care Providers," Centers for Disease Control and Prevention, last reviewed November 10, 2020, https://www.cdc.gov/cancer/preventinfections/providers.htm.

Chapter 4

1. Kathy Caprino, "5 Steps To Speaking Up Powerfully When You Feel You Can't," *Forbes*, May 16, 2018, https://www.forbes.com /sites/kathycaprino/2018/05/16/5-steps-to-speaking-up -powerfully-when-you-feel-you-cant/?sh=2d6b6b086517.

2. Joanne Buzaglo, Ph.D., "Empowering Patients to Become Effective Self-Advocates," *Psychology Today*, November 17, 2016, https:// www.psychologytoday.com/us/blog/the-patient-s-voice/201611 /empowering-patients-become-effective-self-advocates.

3. Kathleen M. Mazor, et al., "Toward Patient-Centered Cancer Care: Patient Perceptions of Problematic Events, Impact, and Response," *Journal of Clinical Oncology* 30 no. 15 (May 20, 2012), 1784-1790, doi.org/10.1200/JCO.2011.38.1384.

4. Kimberly A Fisher, et al., "We want to know: patient comfort speaking up about breakdowns in care and patient experience," *BMJ Quality & Safety* 28 no. 1 (2019), 190-197, dx.doi.org/10.1136 /bmjqs-2018-008159.

Chapter 5

1. Office for Civil Rights, "Your Rights Under HIPAA," U.S. Department of Health & Human Services, November 2, 2020, https://www.hhs.gov/hipaa/for-individuals/guidance-materials-for-consumers/index.html?language=es.

2. "AHIMA Consumer Health Information Bill of Rights," American Health Information Management Association, https://library.ahima.org/PdfView?oid=107674.

Chapter 6

1. Markham Heid, "9 Questions Your Doctor Wishes You'd Ask," *Time,* August 30, 2016, https://time.com/4433153/9-questions-ask-doctor/.

2. Kristen G. Engel, MD, et al., "Patient Comprehension of Emergency Department Care and Instructions: Are Patients Aware of When They Do Not Understand?," *Annals of Emergency Medicine,* 53 no. 4 (April 1, 2009), 454-461, doi.org/10.1016/j.annemergmed.2008.05.016.

3. Marra G. Katz, et al., "Patient Literacy and Question-asking Behavior During the Medical Encounter: A Mixed-methods Analysis," *J Gen Intern Med* 22 no. 6 (June 2007), 782-786, doi.org/10.1007/s11606-007-0184-6.

4. Patrick J. Skerrett, "Ask questions to get the most out of a health care visit," Harvard Health Publishing, June 14, 2013, https://www.health.harvard.edu/blog/ask-questions-to-get-the-most-out-of-a-health-care-visit-201306146383.

5. Matthew Hoffman, MD, "A Cancer Diagnosis: What to Do Next?," WebMD, February 13, 2007, https://www.webmd.com/cancer/features/cancer-diagnosis-what-to-do-next#1.

6. "The 10 Questions You Should Know," Agency for Healthcare Research and Quality, November 2020, https://www.ahrq.gov/questions/10questions.html/

Chapter 7

1. "Five things you may not know about second opinions, from the Harvard Health Letter," Harvard Health Publishing, last updated October 7, 2011, https://www.health.harvard.edu/press_releases /five-things-you-may-not-know-about-second-opinions.
2. "Breaking Down the Barriers to a Second Opinion," Johns Hopkins Medicine, Armstrong Institute, April 20, 2017, https:// armstronginstitute.blogs.hopkinsmedicine.org/2017/04/20 /breaking-down-the-barriers-to-a-second-opinion/.

Chapter 8

1. Courtney Porkoláb, "Does Energy Healing Work? Watch 'Healer' Charlie Goldsmith And Decide For Yourself," *Forbes,* November 13, 2017, https://www.forbes.com/sites /courtneyporkolab/2017/11/13/does-energy-healing-work -watch-healer-charlie-goldsmith-and-decide-for-yourself/?sh =29bc6ce22e1f.

Chapter 9

1. "Dumb Things People Say to People With Cancer," Cure, August 2, 2017, https://www.curetoday.com/view/dumb-things -people-say-to-people-with-cancer.
2. Robin Abrahams, "A friend shared her cancer diagnosis on Facebook. How can I offer support?," *The Boston Globe*, June 26, 2018, https://www.bostonglobe.com/magazine/2018/06/26 /friend-shared-her-cancer-diagnosis-facebook-how-can -offer-support/REAobF2RNAoV2uq1rmNn2H/story.html.
3. Diana Mapes, "'Coming out' with cancer: Patients, experts discuss ins and outs of sharing a diagnosis," Fred Hutch, January 8, 2016, https://www.fredhutch.org/en/news/center-news/2016/01 /coming-out-with-cancer-disclosing-diagnosis.html.

4. "How to Tell a Child That a Parent Has Cancer," American Cancer Society, last revised December 20, 2016, https://www.cancer.org /treatment/children-and-cancer/when-a-family-member-has -cancer/dealing-with-diagnosis/how-to-tell-children.html.

Chapter 10

1. James R. Doty, MD, "Why Kindness Heals," HuffPost, January 26, 2016, https://www.huffpost.com/entry/why-kindness-heals _b_9082134.
2. "The Healing Power of Kindness," Dignity Health, https://www .dignityhealth.org/hello-humankindness/power-of-compassion /the-healing-power-of-kindness.

Chapter 11

1. Susan Krauss Whitbourne, Ph.D., "10 Ways to Feel Better About How You Look," *Psychology Today,* July 26, 2014, https://www .psychologytoday.com/us/blog/fulfillment-any-age/201407 /10-ways-feel-better-about-how-you-look.
2. Nicole Spector, "Smiling can trick your brain into happiness— and boost your health," NBC News, last updated January 9, 2018, https://www.nbcnews.com/better/health/smiling-can-trick -your-brain-happiness-boost-your-health-ncna822591.
3. http://lookgoodfeelbetter.org/.
4. "Working During Cancer Treatment," American Cancer Society, last revised May 13, 2019, https://www.cancer.org /treatment/finding-and-paying-for-treatment/understanding -financial-and-legal-matters/working-during-and-after-treatment /working-during-cancer-treatment.html.
5. Deborah Thomas, "4 tips for exercising during cancer treatment," MD Anderson Cancer Center, July 16, 2014, https://www .mdanderson.org/cancerwise/four-tips-for-exercising-during -cancer-treatment.h00-158910123.html.

Chapter 12

1. "Feelings and Cancer," National Cancer Institute, last updated August 20, 2018, https://www.cancer.gov/about-cancer/coping /feelings.
2. Shoba Sreenivasan, Ph.D. and Linda E. Weinberger, Ph.D., "Do You Believe in Miracles?," *Psychology Today*, December 15, 2017, https://www.psychologytoday.com/us/blog/emotional -nourishment/201712/do-you-believe-in-miracles.

Chapter 13

1. Matthew Hoffman, MD, "A Cancer Diagnosis: What to Do Next?," WebMD, February 13, 2007, https://www.webmd.com /cancer/features/cancer-diagnosis-what-to-do-next#1.
2. Lisa Stein, "Living with Cancer: Eight Things You Need to Know," *Scientific American*, July 16, 2008, https://www.scientific american.com/article/living-with-cancer-8-things/.

Acknowledgments

This book was much harder to write than my first. Going back and revisiting one of the hardest times of my life and sifting through painful memories to pull out the learnings was way more difficult than I thought it would be. Some days I was not so sure that capturing my experiences, even if someone else could learn from them, was something I wanted to do. But each time someone asked me about the book and I shared a part of the learning journey, they responded in ways that let me know I should continue.

More thanks than words can acknowledge go out to my husband, David, who was at my side every step of the way, including every moment of treatment, recovery, and healing. Thanks, and much love, to my mom, who was always there with her presence, strength, nursing expertise, and healing, homemade food. My kids, Jake and Ellie, went about life with strength and normalcy, giving me strength and normalcy. Dear friends Merry, DeAnn, Nanette, Ella, and Kristin took great care of me with frequent and beautiful gifts and meals. Lisa gave me direction, guidance, and great advice from someone who had lived through cancer herself.

To the colectomy surgery team at UPMC Presbyterian Hospital, led by Dr. Kenneth Lee; all the nurses, especially oncology nurses

Leslie and Amanda; and all the medical team members who cared for me along my journey, thank you. Alik, bless you for helping to heal my energy.

My fellow "warriors" and survivor friends, whose stories are included in this book, deserve thanks from the heart. So many of these other survivors have suffered greatly and, despite so much pain, have shared their stories so others can learn and gain different perspectives. Thank you from the bottom of my heart to those who so unselfishly shared their touching personal stories and wisdom—Sylvia, Stacy, Lisa, Andrea, Susan, Ovie, Liz, Anna, Marie, Stacy H., and Brandie—and thanks to the many others who shared experiences that helped shape this book.

Brooke Warner of She Writes Press helped to set the book on a course for publishing. Elizabeth Kracht, a freelance editor and literary agent at Kimberly Cameron & Associates, provided thoughtful, professional, and much-appreciated personal perspective editing to turn the idea of a manuscript into a book.

To anyone who asked how I was doing, sent a card, sent food, conveyed his or her feelings, reached out via Facebook or family, or asked how the book was coming, you'll never know how much a simple, kind gesture means to someone who is recovering from cancer. Even when you really don't know what to say or do, a small act of kindness really does matter.

About the Author

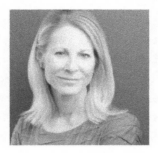

Kelley Skoloda is a wife, mom, daughter, sister, aunt, author, MBA, the founder and CEO of KS Consulting & Capital, an angel investor, and, now, a cancer survivor. Her family is the center of her life, and she loves to golf, cook, travel, and enjoy cat humor with them. Kelley loves being her own boss and started her own business just six months prior to being diagnosed with cancer. She is amazed by how her family, life, and work all survived and thrived through her cancer journey.

A sought-after marketing consultant by day, Kelley works with clients to communicate better with their female audiences. In the mornings and evenings, she connects women-led start-ups to angel funding and is an investor and co-chair of the Investment Committee for the Next Act Fund. She spent many years as a partner at a major public relations firm, where she ran the global brand marketing practice and cultivated a robust network of industry contacts.

Kelley is an influential voice on marketing to women from the page to the stage. Her business book, *Too Busy to Shop: Marketing to Multi-Minding Women*, was named a "must read" by Publishers Weekly and is carried on Amazon. Kelley has spoken at global venues, including the Consumer Electronics Show, M2W, Marketing to Gen Z, Swipe Right, and the PRSA International Conference. Recently, she and her son, Jake, a nineteen-year old student and president of the Millennial Ad Network, have been speaking at events on the topic of generational entrepreneurism.

Kelley has been named one of the "most influential women in business" by the *Pittsburgh Post-Gazette* and has been voted into the PRSA Pittsburgh Hall of Fame. She currently serves on the UPMC Children's Hospital of Pittsburgh Foundation Board of Trustees and the Excela Health Board of Directors and has previously served on the BlogHer/SheKnows and the Seton Hill University boards of trustees and as a member of The *Today* Show Parenting Network.

Skoloda has been quoted and her work has been featured in HuffPost, Time.com, Today.com, Fortune.com, *Forbes*, *Adweek*, Brandweek, C-SPAN, and many other media outlets.

Kelley is grateful every day for the love and support she received throughout her health challenges. She has newfound pleasure in the simple things in life—a great cup of coffee in the morning, a beautiful sky, the love of her family and close friends, and time spent together.

Author photo © Michael Cavotta

SELECTED TITLES FROM SHE WRITES PRESS

She Writes Press is an independent publishing company founded to serve women writers everywhere. Visit us at www.shewritespress.com.

Hug Everyone You Know: A Year of Community, Courage, and Cancer by Antoinette Truglio Martin. $16.95, 978-1-63152-262-8. Cancer is scary enough for the brave, but for a wimp like Antoinette Martin, it was downright terrifying. With the help of her community, however, Martin slowly found the courage within herself to face cancer—and to do so with perseverance and humor.

The Longest Mile: A Doctor, a Food Fight, and the Footrace that Rallied a Community Against Cancer by Christine Meyer, MD. $16.95, 978-1-63152-043-3. In a moment of desperation, after seeing too many patients and loved ones battle cancer, a doctor starts running team—never dreaming what a positive impact it will have on her community.

Body 2.0: Finding My Edge Through Loss and Mastectomy by Krista Hammerbacher Haapala. An authentic, inspiring guide to reframing adversity that provides a new perspective on preventative mastectomy, told through the lens of the author's personal experience.

Stay, Breathe with Me: The Gift of Compassionate Medicine by Helen Allison, RN, MSW with Irene Allison. $16.95, 978-1-63152-062-4. From the voices of the seriously ill, their families, and a specialist with a lifelong experience in caring for them comes the wisdom of a person-centered approach—one that brings heart and compassion back into health care.

The Vitamin Solution: Two Doctors Clear the Confusion about Vitamins and Your Health by Dr. Romy Block and Dr. Arielle Levitan. $17.95, 978-1-63152-014-3. Drs. Romy Block and Arielle Levitan cut through all of the conflicting data about vitamins to provide readers with a concise, medically sound approach to vitamin use as a means of feeling better and enhancing health.

The Self-Care Solution: A Modern Mother's Must-Have Guide to Health and Well-Being by Julie Burton. $16.95, 978-1-63152-068-6. Full of essential physical, emotional and relational self-care tools—and based on research by the author that includes a survey of hundreds of moms—this book is a life raft for moms who often feel like they are drowning in the sea of motherhood.

www.ingramcontent.com/pod-product-compliance
Lightning Source LLC
Chambersburg PA
CBHW020932280625
28807CB00003B/24